Also, by Chuks I. Ndukwe
Available everywhere

The Courage To Aspire
A MATTER OF FAITH
THE AUDACITY OF DESTINY

NAKED COMPASSION

To Give Her A Break

Chuks I. Ndukwe

What Readers Say About
NAKED COMPASSION

I found "NAKED COMPASSION" very interesting, and I enjoyed reading it. If this book were around when I was growing up, most of my friends would not be in the situation they find themselves in these days. I encourage everybody of childbearing age to read this book

~ C. Geter

If you ever tried to talk to your children about birth control and watched your daughters roll their eyes and boys come at you with "I don't want to hear about birth control attitude," you will appreciate NAKED COMPASSION. My message for young people who hate condoms and can't afford to have a baby is to read this book and learn how to uncomplicate your life.

~ R. Davis

I was surprised to learn from this book that the government ranked the pullout among traditional birth control. Knowing that the pullout has no side effects and costs nothing makes it highly attractive. I believe young people will save themselves lots of trouble by learning how to pull out successfully. For me, any birth control that requires the active participation of men and women gets my vote.

~D. Small

As a believer in women's right to choose, the smart pullout expands the range of birth control women can choose. NAKED COMPASSION can be one of the most impactful books in reducing unwanted pregnancy if young people avail themselves of its lessons.

~J. Kruba

Every parent knows how hard it is to discuss sex and birth control with their kids. But now, they can buy NAKED COMPASSION, drop it on the kid's lap, and walk away without saying a word. The subtitle, "To Give Her A Break," is undoubtedly the point of this book. I met the author when he was attending Northeastern University in Boston. Over the years, we built trust and memory that will last a lifetime, and I credit this book's content for our enduring friendship.

The endearing part of this book is that the author is preaching what he has practiced since he was seventeen. I am delighted that Chuks has written a book that allows people to avoid unwanted pregnancy, child support woes, and raising a child they cannot afford. And still prevent toxic substances from getting into the woman's body.

~ J. Marshall

Naked Compassion: To Give Her A Break.

Published by:
Ikebiebooks

Ikebiebooks Publishing

info@ikebiebooks.com

ISBN-13: 978-0-9990705-3-6 (Paperback)
ISBN-10: 0-9990705-3-3

ISBN-13: 978-0-9990705-4-3 (Ebook)
ISBN-10: 0-9990705-4-1

Library of Congress Control Number: 2018817424

Contents

Contents

Contents

Contents

Contents

Contents

Introduction

✳ ✳ ✳

Imagine a life where you can enjoy a passionate sexual relationship without worrying about unwanted pregnancy, sexually transmitted infections, and life-threatening birth control side effects.

Of all the gifts a man can give the woman he loves: flowers, lingerie, diamond, silver, and gold. I can't think of anything more precious than lifting the burden of unwanted pregnancy off her shoulders and taking an active role. It frees her mind from all unwanted pregnancy-related fears. It engenders trust, fosters a happy relationship, allows her to enjoy the peace of mind she deserves and empowers her to exercise her femininity as she pleases. Very often, this act of compassion lays the foundation for a happy and lasting relationship.

Most unwanted pregnancies happen by accident when we least think of it or are absorbed in the euphoria of sexual pleasure. In some cases, it starts with a casual flirtatious Hi! Sometimes, it progresses to dating. Occasionally people meet and jump right into bed, and the male hopes the lady uses some birth control and the type she chooses feels good.

The tough choice of birth control becomes a significant task for her unless she is already familiar with different methods. Whatever method she chooses poses some health risks—side effects that do not worry boys. So she settles on her birth control method of choice, and then they enjoy precious time together and fulfil their sexual needs. The thought of what comes next or the fear of the unexpected always lingers until the next period.

Naked Compassion

Then the never-ending cycle starts all over again. In some other cases, mates become complaisant and plunge right into sexual activities without the thought of unwanted pregnancy and fear of possible sexually transmitted infection.

There are different birth control methods in use today with varying results. Most of these methods come with high financial costs and devastating side effects. When you combine the monetary price with the value of the incidental side effects they bring about, the mere thought of adopting any one of them becomes a big deal—a frightening decision with drastic consequences.

A friend of mine asked me: "can you believe how they force women to choose birth control methods based on which one's benefit outweighs its risks and disadvantages?" Her statement is a sad commentary that offers women no comfort or peace of mind. Further, it exposes the inadequacy of educators' and scientists' work in educating and informing women of all available birth control methods.

Of all the birth control methods available today, there's one and only one kind (withdrawal method) that does not cost a dime, does not have any side effects and is safe and effective. However, one must know how one's reproductive system works, and the body's different degrees of sensitivity during sexual intercourse. It requires thoughtfulness, dedication, consistency, motivated caring, and compassion.

This book is all about inspiring, empowering, and teaching people how to practice the best birth control (unwanted pregnancy prevention) method that gets the job done and makes you feel safe, happy, and worry-free in the end.

Additionally, it aims at reducing, if not eliminating, the fear of abortion from every woman's mind, providing men with the

Introduction

knowledge they need to help them take an active and leading role in preventing unwanted pregnancy and reducing the fear of sexually transmitted infections.

Using this book as your guide for birth control or pregnancy prevention techniques, you will learn non-medical facts about your reproductive system. You will better know what is going on when you have sex, how the intensity of the body's sensitive nerves change, and how to pull out your penis from the vagina before ejaculation. Everybody's fantasy is to continue having fun after sex—talking, teasing, cuddling, telling stories, and falling asleep in each other's arms instead of fearing getting pregnant. This book helps you realize that fantasy.

First, you must stop thinking about sex casually and realize it is vital to healthy living. By that, I mean: You have to understand what is going on when you have sex and understand it accounts for your happiness, body fitness, and tranquility of mind and soul. Why not do it right and have a baby only when you want one without overloading the woman's body with pills or unhealthy toxic substances?

If you are truly serious about safe birth control or unwanted pregnancy prevention, you need to shake off your casual attitude towards sex and take a hard look at the challenge. This statement isn't thrown at you to discourage you. Still, instead, it's to get you raved up to learn the lessons in this book and enjoy the pleasant experience of lovemaking and its full benefits without being burdened by the fear of pregnancy you've not planned.

Friends and relatives will say a few things to discourage you and fuel your doubt. Religious beliefs will undoubtedly play their part. As usual, cultural mores, peer perception, and less-than-honest medical opinions will pull your mind in different

Naked Compassion

directions.

However, here's the question: Whose life is on the line here? What sense does it make to stick to an undoubtedly dangerous and life-threatening practice instead of one that is safe, effective, and lets you have total control?

Because of men's cavalier attitude towards pregnancy, Naked Compassion contains many discussions about conception, pregnancy, and women's pregnancy intentions.

However, to a more significant extent, it is all about a man's genuine and discernible compassion, understanding the burden every woman bears to protect against unwanted pregnancy and how to take an active role in alleviating her burden.

As I grapple with writing this book, I wonder why so many girls are obese these days, and a disproportionate number of women are dying of cancer. My fiancé Renee battled cancer for several years before she gave up. Before she died, she told me stories about her battle with birth control side effects before we met. One day on her hospital bed, she pulled me down on her chest, sobbed, and said, "I don't think I'd be lying here, staring death in the face if we had met before I started using toxic birth control." Her frail voice pierced through my heart and made me feel guilty though there was nothing I could do to change her condition at the time. Whenever I think of women who have died of cancer like her and others with cancer today, I wonder what part birth control plays in their plight.

I do not intend this book to be controversial. Instead, I want to share my experience and encourage other men to realize that helping ease their mate's unwanted pregnancy concerns will likely infuse unbelievable happiness and staying power into their relationships.

PART 1

NAKED

COMPASSION

On Pregnancy

Pregnancy is when the creator transforms the female body into a sacred laboratory of natural wonders.

Conception

It's as though the concept of marriage with but one person at a time stems from that sacred moment after sex when a man's sperm burrows into the woman's egg and locks the door so no other sperm can get in.

✳✳✳

After each successful sexual intercourse, by which I mean one that ends with a healthy orgasm. The male partner releases millions of sperm. This army of sperm begins a race upstream in search of the female egg. In most cases, all of them would not make it to the uterus. In many cases, the ones that do start the final part of the race to find the egg. The race winner is not the first sperm to reach the egg but one that burrows into the egg and locks others out. Although far from other exciting material we love to immerse ourselves in, it is essential to understand the pathways and journey the sperm makes within the woman's reproductive system before fertilizing the woman's egg to prevent the sperm from starting the race in the first place.

Fertilization

Each month inside a woman's ovaries, a group of eggs grows in tiny fluid-filled sacs called the follicle. Eventually, one of the eggs breaks away from the follicle — usually two weeks before her next period. After the separation, the follicle develops

On Pregnancy

into something called the corpus luteum. The corpus luteum then releases a hormone that helps thicken the lining of the woman's uterus, preparing it for the egg's arrival. After being released, the egg moves into the fallopian tube. Then it waits for about 24 hours to be fertilized by a single sperm. All these happen, on average, about two weeks after her last period. If no sperm fertilizes the egg, it moves through the uterus and disintegrates. Her hormone levels go back to normal. Her body sheds the thick lining of the uterus, and her period starts. However, if one sperm does make its way into the fallopian tube (during sex) and forces itself into the egg, now you have fertilization. At this moment, the sperm that gets in determines her baby's genes and gender at the instant of fertilization. If the sperm has a Y chromosome, her baby will be a boy. If it has an X chromosome, the baby will be a girl.

Pregnancy

Pregnancy is also known as gestation, when one or more offspring develop inside a woman. Pregnancy occurs through sexual intercourse or assisted reproductive technology. Childbirth occurs roughly forty weeks from the last menstrual period—just over nine lunar months, where each month is twenty-nine and a half days. When measured from conception, it's about thirty-eight weeks.

An embryo is a developing offspring during the first eight weeks following conception, after which the embryo becomes a fetus until birth. Pregnancy tests may confirm early pregnancy, and pregnancy symptoms may include:

- Missed periods
- Tender breasts

Naked Compassion

- Hunger
- Nausea and vomiting
- Frequent urination

Pregnancy Trimesters

- The first trimester is weeks one through twelve following fertilization. The fertilized egg moves from the fallopian tube and attaches to the uterus, where it begins to form an embryo and placenta.

- CDC defines the second trimester as week thirteen to twenty-eight of pregnancy; the mother can feel the baby's movement around the middle.

- The third trimester is weeks twenty-nine through forty.

Term pregnancy is thirty-seven through forty-one weeks calibrated as follows:

- Early term— thirty-seven and thirty-eight weeks
- Full-term— thirty-nine and forty weeks
- Late-term— forty-one weeks
- Post-term— after forty-one weeks

By estimation, 213 million pregnancies occurred worldwide in 2012, of which 190 million occurred in developing countries and 23 million in developed countries. Research shows that the number of pregnant women ages 15 to 44 is 133 out of 1,000

On Pregnancy

women who took part in the study. About 10% to 15% of recognized pregnancies ended in miscarriage. In 2013, complications of pregnancy resulted in 293,000 deaths, down from 377,000 deaths in 1990. The common causes of difficulties are:

- Maternal bleeding
- Complications of abortion
- High blood pressure
- Maternal sepsis
- Obstructed labor

Although people celebrate pregnancy as a happy milestone in a woman's life, we must also recognize it as a painful period for those women whose pregnancies came as a surprise—unintended or unwanted. Furthermore, some women are afraid of getting pregnant due to medical or biological reasons; hence, it is essential to separate wanted, unwanted, and mistimed pregnancies, as shown below, because each group's attitude towards pregnancy varies. Here's the classification for better understanding:

- Wanted means the pregnancy occurred at about the time the couple or mother wanted to become pregnant.

- Mistimed by less than two years ("moderately mistimed") means the pregnancy occurred too soon—specifically, less than two years before the mother wanted to become pregnant.

- Mistimed by two years or more ("seriously mistimed") means the pregnancy occurred too soon—specifically, two years or more before the mother wanted to become pregnant.

- Unintended pregnancy means the pregnancy is unexpected (i.e., it occurred when no children or more children were expected).

- Unwanted pregnancy means the mother never wanted a baby or a particular birth order (second, third, fourth).

Wanted Pregnancy

Wanted pregnancies happen at "the right time" or later than the desired period due to infertility or difficulties in conceiving. That means the woman and her mate have been having sex with the expectation of having a child. The following are a few ways of determining wanted pregnancy:

- Mates are having sex without contraceptive methods or fear of having a baby.

- The couple has been seeking fertility help

- Mates have planned it and are able and willing to parent the baby

- The couple is eager to find prenatal care

- Mates are excited to usher the baby into the world.

- Mates spend undue time comparing the baby's look to either.

- Mates are eager to show off the baby

On Pregnancy

Unintended pregnancy

Unintended pregnancies are unexpected (i.e., they occur when no children, or no more children, were expected). Another concept related to unintended pregnancy is an unplanned pregnancy, which happens when the woman gets pregnant because she forgot to use any birth control method. The usual methods of measuring unintended pregnancy reflect a woman's intentions before becoming pregnant.

The concept of unintended pregnancy has helped governments study human populations' characteristics, especially regarding size, density, growth, distribution, migration, and their impact on social and economic conditions in understanding fertility. It also helps public health practitioners prevent unplanned childbearing and help women determine whether and when to have children.

Researchers believe that accurate measurement of pregnancy intentions is vital in understanding fertility-related behavior, forecasting fertility, and estimating the unmet need for contraception. It facilitates comprehension of pregnancy intentions' impact on maternal and child health, designing family planning programs, evaluating their effectiveness, and creating and evaluating community-based programs that prevent unintended pregnancies.

To a more significant extent, the concept of unintended pregnancy is complex. Hence pregnancy intentions are increasingly viewed as encompassing, affective, cognitive, cultural, and contextual. The government's purpose in developing a complete understanding of pregnancy intentions aims to persuade women to use contraceptives to prevent unintended pregnancies and improve women's and their children's health. You can determine unintended pregnancies in the following ways:

- Mates are having sex without contraceptives but are afraid of having a baby

- Mates are having sex with contraceptives, but the woman gets pregnant regardless

- Mates have not planned to have a baby and are neither able nor willing to parent the baby

- Mates are less likely to seek early prenatal care

- Mates are not ready to welcome the baby into the world due to medical, economic, or social reasons

- The couple is not excited about the arrival of the baby

- Couples are less enthusiastic about comparing the baby to either of them

- Couples do not show off their baby

Unwanted Pregnancies

Unwanted pregnancies are those that occur when mothers want no children. It is closely related to unintended pregnancy (described earlier), which happens when the woman uses a contraceptive method, hoping it would protect her from pregnancy, but it doesn't. The usual methods of measuring unwanted pregnancy reflect a woman's intentions before becoming pregnant. Here are a few ways to determine whether a pregnancy is unwanted:

On Pregnancy

- Discernable ambivalence towards conception
- Likelihood of abortion
- Likelihood of miscarriage
- Eager to abandon the baby at birth
- Readiness to give up all maternal responsibilities

Ambivalence towards conception involves emotional and psychological factors that often determine attitude towards sex. Unfortunately, unwanted pregnancy resolutions are often wrongfully grouped because women make them at different ages and stages in their reproductive lives for various biological, emotional, and medical reasons.

Different studies have found that the cause of fear of engaging in sexual intercourse is often different from childbearing concerns. Childbearing concerns may emerge after a woman has experienced her first birth. The following anecdotes illustrate the difference between childbearing fears and ambivalence towards sexual intercourse.

Sexual Ambivalence

I met Patricia while we were attending Northeastern University in Boston. She was beautiful and loved to dance mostly with girls because she felt uncomfortable holding hands with men. We went out clubbing once on a Saturday night. Many familiar faces were dancing on the floor, a few lived on my block, but Patricia lived further away. I had a car, so I gave Patricia and three of her friends a ride at the end of the night. Then we became friends and went out together regularly. We grew close only to the point of dancing together—without touching each other. A few months later, Pat invited me over for dinner.

After dinner, we spent the evening reminiscing about different clubs we love and the atmosphere that makes a club inviting. We also talked about our friends; how awkward she feels dancing with most of them, then she joked about how I'd sit there until she dragged me out of my seat to dance with her even though I had no problem asking other girls for a dance. "Why is that?" She joked. Then a few months later, she invited herself to my apartment after club hours.

When we got to my apartment, the time was about three-thirty in the morning, so we sat on the couch and chatted for the remainder of the night, and then I gave her a ride home. As I turned to go back home, she signaled me to pack. So I packed the car and waited to hear why she signaled me to pack the car.

"Pack the car and come in for breakfast," she said. So I packed the car, went inside her apartment, prepared two scrambled eggs, tea, and toast, and ate breakfast together before I left. None of us had a telephone in our apartments, so we communicated in person in the street, at the school campus, or occasionally rang each other's doorbell.

The next time we went out, Patricia told everybody that she had spent Saturday night with me. "We had a pretty good time preparing breakfast together," she said. That hit everybody like a bullet. "Say what?" Richard asked as his eyes almost popped out of their sockets and others sat in what seemed like uncomfortable silence because Patricia disliked men.

After that weekend, Patricia and I became chums. She'd drag me out to the floor inside the club, and we'd dance to slow

On Pregnancy

music, holding hands. Then after club hours, I'd drop everybody off before taking her home. Sometimes we spent the night telling each other stories about our childhood—how we snuck out and did things our parents would have killed us for—if they knew. However, still unknown was why she decided to dance intimately with a man suddenly.

One night she opened up, "I hate men. They are evil, but you are different—you are kind, respectful, and gentle." "Why do you hate men?" I asked. She sobbed and told me that her stepfather sexually abused her at the tender age of ten. So men's touch makes her skin crawl. I was so horrified by Patricia's revelation that I probed no further. Instead, I hugged her and told her I was sorry for what had happened to her. In this case, Pat's sexual ambivalence and repulsion from men resulted from her early life experience.

Fear of Childbearing

Sharon lives across the street from me. Along with her petite stature, she's provocatively seductive. So much so that Sharon once attracted the attention of a passing-by police officer. She immediately accosted the officer for looking at her while coming home from the store. Because of Sharon's attitude, men find her intimidating and challenging to approach. But on a very personal level, she's kind and generous. However, I did not know it at the time. At this moment, my world was collapsing, so I worked all day, all week, and I had only seen her on a few occasions when I was off from work. On those few occasions, when I stood by my window looking outside, I could see her stunning looks and sent out my unspoken compliments.

One day, I was on my way to the police headquarters in Newark, New Jersey, to do a fingerprint and background check

Naked Compassion

for my insurance certificate application. The office is at the center of the city, and there is no free parking space around the office building. So I made a quick stop at the pizza shop on the ground floor of my apartment building for a few minutes to get quarters to feed the parking meter.

Sharon grabbed my attention as she has always done. But I had no time to talk to her, so I ignored her and turned around, attempting to leave. Suddenly she said, "I thought you came to the shop to buy me a slice of pizza."

"Are you talking to me?" I asked.

"Yes, Mister, I am talking to you," she replied.

"Sorry, remind me next time you see me; I'm running late," I replied and left.

A few days later, Sharon and I met again in the lobby of my apartment building when she came to see her aunt. I remembered the last time we met and bought her a slice of pizza I had promised her.

Walking away, she asked, "Oh, you remember the slice of pizza you promised me? Thank you." Then this, "Are you that stupid to not know when a girl is flirting with you or simply too stuck up to give me your telephone number, or am I not pretty enough for you?"

"I think you are stunning but too young for me," I answered.

"You are crazy, Mister," she said and showed me her ID card to prove she was twenty-seven years old. Finally, I gave her my telephone number.

So shortly after that episode, she called me, and then we began to talk on the phone for a while before she visited me. On her first visit, I served some drinks, and then we talked about the

On Pregnancy

day I saw her accosting a police officer. "That was some shit," she said, "that popo has no business looking at a woman like that." Now we became friends to the point she'd buzz me up whenever she saw my lights on. I liked Sharon a lot, especially her sense of sarcasm and constant jabs at everything I said. I did not react to her seductive and friendly jokes, provoking curious mockery for a while. So one day, she joked, "most men don't let pretty girls lean on them without letting their hands wander all over her. I guess you are different."

"I only cross a bridge built on a strong foundation," I said.

"That's beautiful; I guess we have time to find out what you mean by that," she replied.

On Saturday evening—the first time we went out, she took me to meet her father, auntie, and uncle before we went out for dinner at Red Lobster restaurant. As we sat down to wait for our order, she began to ask me a series of questions, one of which was why I was single. So I turned the table and asked her why a pretty girl like herself did not have a boyfriend.

Sharon paused for a few seconds. Then she said, "I am looking for a real man like you, but he is hard to find,"

"What makes a real man?" I asked.

"A real man does not drool over a pretty girl at first sight, nor crowd her space, call her a million times—day and night, and jump all over her and ask her for a relationship," she said. "Every time I like a man, the first thing he does is ask me to be his girlfriend without taking time to know me, then he'll go on and talk about marriage and how many children he wants and stalk me if I say no."

"So, aside from the stalking part, what's wrong with that?" I asked.

"I cannot bear children," she said. "The doctor told me I

could not have a child due to abnormal pelvis. I am afraid of getting pregnant." Then she began to lament the use of birth control.

"I have a serious problem already," she said, "how can somebody expect me to put more shit in my body as if my mother raised a fool? If any man wants my love, he must wear some rubber."

In this case, Sharon enjoys sex and wants to have a permanent boyfriend but is adamantly afraid of getting pregnant.

The most crucial fact about Sharon's view is not the agony of not having a child, which is heart-wrenching and deserving of sympathy. But her antipathy to all manner of traditional birth control is because of the side effects that cause countless women immense suffering they would not otherwise suffer.

Sharon is not alone in her views because thousands of women in the United States and millions worldwide share the same plight. So from the perspective of the right to pursue happiness, women like Sharon deserve sympathy.

A sense of empathy for women like Sharon and avoidance of not-so-enjoyable feelings men experience while having sex with a condom makes this book "Naked Compassion" one of its time's conscience-shaping books. Because it helps men enjoy sex and women avoid the side effects of traditional birth control.

The fear of childbearing and sexual ambivalence is biological for many women, and they deserve exceptional attention.

Age Income and Racial Factors

According to another study published in 2006, 49% of

On Pregnancy

pregnancies were unintended, and 48% in 2001. Among women 19 years and younger, more than 4 out of 5 pregnancies were unexpected or unwanted.

The proportion of unintended pregnancies was highest among girls younger than 15, at 98%. Between 2001 and 2006, unintended pregnancies declined from 89% to 79% among teens aged 15–17. It increased from 79% to 83% among women 18 and 19 and from 59% to 64% among women 20–24.

Significant increases in unintended pregnancy rates were among women with lower education, low income, and cohabiting women. In addition, recent National Survey of Family Growth data shows a fewer decline in the overall unintended births between the 1982 and the 2006–2010 surveys. Women who were more likely to experience unexpected or unwanted births include:

1. Unmarried women.

2. Black women.

3. Less-educated women

4. Less income-earning women.

The United States family planning goals aim to improve pregnancy planning and spacing and prevent unintended pregnancy. So the objective is to increase the proportion of wanted or intended pregnancies to 56%. Family planning can reduce unwanted or unintended pregnancies by expanding access to effective, longer-acting, reversible contraceptive methods.

Naked Compassion

Public Health Consideration

The government reviewed studies on unwanted pregnancies to lay a scientific foundation for public health efforts and prevent unintended pregnancies from September 1999 to May 2001. The following topics are a part of that review of the Center for Disease Control's strategic planning activities.

- How different cultures perceive fertility, relationships, and sexuality among different groups of women worldwide.

- How women of different educational backgrounds view and think about sexuality, relationships, and pregnancy.

- How women of different economic statuses: poor, middle-class, and wealthy women, think about sexuality, relationships, and pregnancy.

- How women of different experiences express their sexuality and views ab

- out accessibility to their favorite birth control means.

PART 2

NAKED
COMPASSION

On Birth Control Methods

One of my favorite moments is when a guy, at that certain point in a relationship, says something desperately hopeful like, 'Are you on the pill?' I simply say, 'No, are you?

~ Roxane Gay

Naked Compassion

Common Problem

If the world were merely seductive, that would be easy. If it were merely challenging, that would be no problem. But I arise in the morning with a desire to improve the world and enjoy the world. This makes it hard to plan the day.

~ E. B. White

***

In dealing with problems, one must consider the nature of the problem and ask a few questions: is the problem an economic, financial, technological, scientific, or social problem? If the relevant issue is a social problem, then the next logical follow-up questions are, what is the case's nature? Is it physical, mental, behavioral, or biological?

Ask these questions because experts can handle each problem differently with varying effectiveness and results. The problem we are dealing with in this book is social—unwanted pregnancy, the cause of which is a man filling the woman's vagina with semen.

Looking beyond the joy of welcoming a baby into the world, the couple's gratification of knowing that they are blessed with fertility—if it's their first, unwanted pregnancy and childbirth poses severe problems in different ways to governments, families, and individuals. In some countries experiencing overpopulation, unwanted pregnancy is a

On Birth Control Methods

significant problem that compels political leaders to violate individual sexual liberties, such as: regulating the number of children a couple can have. It also forces the couple to adopt a predetermined birth control method because every government has limited resources to care for its citizens. It's not surprising that some governments do whatever they can to control overpopulation by restricting the number of children each couple can have.

For families, the cost of raising children can be pretty expensive. When coupled with the cost of education, the number of children the family can handle becomes a significant part of their economic and financial planning. Pregnancy is an essential item on the daily not-to-do list for individuals struggling for advancement in the workplace and sexual liberty because it adversely affects their living standards and professional growth. It can also impact on-time graduation or force a girl to drop out of school altogether for those still in school.

In many under-developed countries where cultural values transcend everything, society frowns upon unwanted pregnancy; hence, pregnancy avoidance is the number one birth control.

Attitudes and behaviors of male partners often determine how much the female partner considers pregnancy a problem. On the other hand, the female partner's views and whether she is suitable for marriage determines how much her getting pregnant is a problem for her male partner. Pregnancy can be a problem for both males and females, except when a couple or a woman wants the pregnancy and is willing, able, and ready to welcome her baby into the world.

Sexual intercourse occurs more frequently outside of marriage and committed relationships. Unplanned pregnancy has increased in virtually all developed countries. So it is unsurprising that the demand for birth control pills and other methods keeps growing.

Common Solution

As is always the case, common problems require a standard solution. As in the case of problem determination, for a problem solver to come up with the most desirable solution, he must ask himself a few questions: Is there more than one solution for the underlying problem? If so, which solution is most discernably effective? Is this attractive solution also affordable so that even the community's poorest can avail themselves of it? Is it as safe as it is effective? Is it a preventive or corrective measure? Is it easy enough to apply? If not, how can the affected learn how to use the solution?

Another question is, how does the solution affect the lives of those involved? Does it adversely affect the experience or the standard of living of those applying it? If not, to what extent is it life-enhancing or advantageous? However, suppose it adversely affects those using it. In that case, we have a different line of questioning: to what extent is it life-threatening or disadvantageous?

In the case of unwanted pregnancy, the universally accepted solution is contraception or birth control. Some of these birth control methods do not work as advertised, and others create unintended problems for those who use them because they lack awareness of other safer options. For that reason, Naked Compassion seeks to transform withdrawal into awareness-based birth control women can embrace because it is practical, safe, life-enhancing, and poses no side effects.

On Birth Control Methods

According to a report commissioned by CDC and Family Planning Services, birth control prevents about 1.3 million unintended pregnancies annually in the United States. Sterilization has markedly decreased pregnancy rates. Modern contraceptives are highly efficient; many American women are still concerned about their side effects and are unhappy about the limited birth control types available. "Despite considerable progress, we do not know how pregnancy intentions affect the use of contraceptives," the report said. The following factors affect women's failure to practice contraception:

- Negative attitudes about the methods

- Increased perceived barriers to method use;

- Perceived low support from partners and peers;

- Poor communication skills;

- Indulging in risky behavior;

For teenagers residing in neighborhoods characterized by inadequate supervision, the cause of women's failure to practice contraception is insufficient community resources and behaviors that depart from a healthy lifestyle (e.g., dropping out of school). Increasing concerns about sexually transmitted infections, including HIV, play an essential role in understanding why people choose contraceptives. Also, eagerness to prevent infection and unwanted pregnancy makes it easy for women to adopt a barrier method. Women who use a condom to protect against disease and pregnancy use the technique more consistently than others.

Undoubtedly, man's involvement in the process of human reproduction—conception, pregnancy, and birth is his sperm donation. The significant burden of this process is solely that of a woman to bear. The enzymes, biochemical, protein, sugar, and vital minerals that form, protect, and grow her fetus are integral parts of the woman's body.

Having been around women with different health concerns during pregnancies and having lost my fiancée to breast cancer, if there is a discussion about pregnancy, it is how to ensure the pregnant woman wanted the pregnancy in the first place. And then ensure that she is adequately cared for medically, physically, mentally, and emotionally during her pregnancy. Because a healthy mother is more likely than not to have a healthy baby and a healthy baby is a healthy citizen of a healthy nation.

Until scientists can grow a baby in a tube outside the women's womb, we can reasonably assume that every human being is a woman's product and deserves proper respect and appreciation. The easiest way for a man to demonstrate his consideration and affection is to engage in sexual activities with compassion and understanding and actively assist his mate in preventing unwanted pregnancy.

Unmarried Men and Birth Control

The National Center for Health Statistics surveyed about 3,700 unmarried men. The report found that more men are using male contraception, such as withdrawal during sexual intercourse, in the past three months of the survey.

The study conducted in 2002 found that only 52 percent of the men surveyed said they had used the withdrawal method, condom, or a vasectomy when they last had sex. Currently, that

On Birth Control Methods

number has gone up to 59 percent, and the increase appears among those who reported using withdrawal, as rates of condom and vasectomy use held steady.

In the above study, any female contraceptive method comprises every type, including those used by men and their female partners, while any male contraceptive covers vasectomy, withdrawal, and a condom. Also, among the unmarried men between 15 and 19, 26 percent were likely to practice withdrawal birth control, whereas only 23 percent of those who had never married practiced withdrawal. That means that over sixty percent of the population does not know the effectiveness of withdrawal as a birth control method.

However, these rates remain consistent among whites, blacks, and Hispanics—the three racial groups measured in the study. There is a significant statistical difference in withdrawal rates between never-married men and cohabitating and formerly married men. Among couples who correctly use the withdrawal every time they have sex, the chance of women getting pregnant is only about 4 out of 100. However, it requires a great deal of self-awareness, self-control, and trust between partners.

Therefore, it is challenging to do it correctly during every sexual intercourse. Men must completely pull out of their partner's vagina when sex starts to feel the best. According to another report, about 27 out of 100 women will get pregnant among typical couples who use withdrawal.

Other studies reveal that condom use is likely to result in 18 out of 100, while about nine out of 100 women who use the contraceptive pill will get pregnant in a year. Several such reports indicate that the use of the withdrawal is increasing rapidly. But the question is, why?

The answer is probably the widespread complaints that birth

control users are dissatisfied with their current methods and want something different and safer.

There are other reasons; women feel unhappy about choosing between a permanent form of birth control and a barrier birth control method that they know may blunt sexual pleasure. But this feeling isn't a new phenomenon. Because in part, the cultural acceptance—especially among female partners—of withdrawal as a legitimate birth control method is growing.

In 2014, a study on birth control surveying women of reproductive age found that one out of three women had used the withdrawal at least once in the past month of the research and considered it a backup form of contraception because they were also taking the pill or using other methods. The survey found the same to be true of the men. This survey asks only about male forms of contraception and not about any kind of birth control their female partner may be using.

Types of Birth Control

No, you can't deny women their fundamental rights and pretend it's about your 'religious freedom.' If you don't like birth control, don't use it. Religious freedom doesn't mean you can force others to live by your own beliefs.

~ President Barack Obama

This section contains the different birth control methods women use worldwide and their side effects, costs, and associated legal cases.

Physics reminds us that every action has an equal and

On Birth Control Methods

opposite reaction. Medicine informs us that every drug has side effects. Civics tells us that every legislation has unintended consequences. So we can reasonably surmise that everything comes with a price in life. The following are questions a woman should think about before deciding to adopt any birth control method:

- How much can you sacrifice for a product you are unsure of its safety and efficacy?

- How much pain are you willing to endure from what you are taking to prevent another you do not wish to have?

Undoubtedly, most birth control methods come with a very high price, except the withdrawal method, which is free. So it's this battle over the amount to pay, risk to take, and pain to endure when deciding on a birth control method that compels women to make different birth control choices.

This section contains information we found researching this book on birth control methods, efficacy, costs, and side effects.

The choice of birth control you make today could be why you live happily tomorrow.

Birth Control Implant

The birth control implant, also known as Nexplanon, is a tiny, thin rod about a matchstick's size. The implant releases hormones into a woman's body, preventing her from getting pregnant. A nurse or doctor inserts the implant into a woman's arm to protect her from pregnancy for about four years. It's get-it-and-forget-it birth control. The implant releases the hormone progestin to stop her from getting pregnant in the following ways:

- Progestin on a woman's cervix makes the mucus thick, preventing sperm from moving to her fallopian tube. When sperm can't get to a woman's egg, she can't get pregnant.

- Progestin can also stop ovulation, so there's no egg in the fallopian tube for sperm to fertilize.

One of the remarkable things about the implant is that it lasts for a long time—up to 4 years—but it's not permanent. So, If you decide you want to get pregnant, your doctor can take it out. You're able to get pregnant again quickly. The implant is about 99% effective. So, about 1 in 100 women who use Nexplanon will likely get pregnant in a year.

Since the implant is in a woman's arm, she can't forget to take it or misuse it. She must use condoms and implant to help protect her from both pregnancy and STDs.

Implant Side Effects

"Some women experience side effects after getting Nexplanon, but many adjust to the implant with a few or no problems," the maker says. "Adverse side effects usually go away after a few months, once a woman's body gets used to her implant."

The most common side effect is occasional bleeding or spotting within 12 months. Sometimes the implant causes long-term spotting or a more prolonged and substantial period. However, for most women, the implant causes their periods to

On Birth Control Methods

get lighter. About three out of ten women who undergo the implant stop getting their periods after twelve months. Other uncommon side effects are:

- Headaches
- Breast pain
- Nausea
- Weight gain
- Ovarian cysts
- Discomfort or bruising around the part of the body where the implantation occurred.

Birth Control Pill

Birth control pills are contraceptives with hormones that a woman takes daily to prevent pregnancy. There are many different brands of pills. The capsule is safe, affordable, and works well if you always take it on time. Besides preventing pregnancy, the tablet has many other health benefits. When used correctly, the pill is 99% effective. Realistically, the tablet is about 91% effective because it can be hard to comply with the instructions. So about 9 in 100 women who use the pill will likely get pregnant in twelve months.

However, although tiny, there's the chance that a woman could still get pregnant, even if she takes the tablet according to instructions.

Following the instructions and using the birth control pill correctly gives the woman excellent protection against pregnancy. However, missing or forgetting to take the pills makes it not work.

Women will likely reduce their menstrual cramps, lighten their periods, and reduce their risk of ectopic pregnancy by taking their progestin-only pills according to instructions and prescription. It will also reduce their chance of getting:

- acne
- bone thinning
- the breasts and ovaries cysts
- endometrial and ovarian cancers
- severe ovaries, fallopian tubes, and uterus infections
- iron deficiency (anemia)
- PMS (premenstrual syndrome)

Pill Side Effects

In the same way, like most medications, birth control pills can have side effects. However, most usually go away after two or three months. Many people use the pill with no health problems at all. The rest experience the following side effects:

- The hormones in the pills can change a woman's level of sexual desire.
- She may also bleed between periods and experience sore breasts, headaches, or nausea if she uses progestin-only pills. However, these symptoms go away after three months.

On Birth Control Methods

Birth Control Sponge

The birth control spongy cup is a small, round cup made from soft plastic, which a woman puts deep inside her vagina before having sex. The sponge has a fabric loop to make it easier to take out.

The sponge works if you use it correctly each time during sex. Failure to follow the instructions or use them as directed means the sponge won't work. The sponge is also most effective if you've never given birth before.

Women who have never given birth and use the sponge correctly every time they have sex find it's about 91% effective—that means 9 out of 100 women who use the sponge would get pregnant within a year.

For women who have given birth and always use the sponge correctly every time they have sex, it's about 80% effective—that means that 20 out of 100 sponge users would get pregnant within a year.

Realistically, using the sponge is not easy, so the sponge is 88% effective for women who've never given birth—12 in 100 women who use the sponge and have not given birth before will likely get pregnant in twelve months. Sponge birth control is efficient for 76 out of 100 women who have given birth—so 24 out of 100 women of the sponge-users who've given birth will get pregnant within a year.

You can put your sponge in place 24 hours before sex, so you don't have to worry about birth control during sex. Furthermore, putting your sponge in place before things get hot and crazy allows you to take care of pregnancy prevention without pausing the action. Once the sponge is in your vagina, you can have sex multiple times for the next 24 hours.

Most women can't feel the sponge once it's in their vagina, and many partners don't feel it during sex. The sponge is soft, squishy, and feels like a vagina, so even partners who notice it usually don't care. Knowing that the sponge will protect you from pregnancy can help you relax and enjoy sex more.

The sponge is a good option for women who prefer non-hormonal birth control or can't use hormones because of medical problems. Also, using the sponge while breastfeeding is safe because it's hormone-free.

Condom

Condoms are thin pouches made of latex, plastic, or lambskin, with which a man can cover his penis during sex and stop sperm from getting into his mate's vagina. Condoms prevent STDs by preventing contact with semen and vaginal fluids and limiting skin-to-skin contact that can spread sexually transmitted infections.

Even if you use different birth control to avoid pregnancy, it's good to use condoms or female condoms every time you have sex to protect yourself from STDs. Condoms work well, if used correctly, every time you have sex, and that means you should keep them in place until you finish having sex. Condoms won't work if you use them occasionally or don't fully cover the penis. Remember to keep a pack of condoms close by before you get busy and use one when the time is right.

IUD

An IUD is a tiny device a woman inserts inside her uterus to

On Birth Control Methods

prevent her from getting pregnant. It is a reversible and effective birth control method. It stands for the Intrauterine device or a device a woman wears inside her uterus. It is a small piece of flexible plastic shaped like a "T." It is also called an IUC—intrauterine contraception. The IUD brands that the FDA has approved in the United States are ParaGard, Mirena, Kyleena, Skyla, and Liletta. These IUDs come in 2 types: copper IUDs (ParaGard) and hormonal IUDs (Mirena, Kyleena, Skyla, and Liletta).

IUDs are about 99% effective. That means fewer than 1 in 100 women who use an IUD will likely become pregnant in twelve months. IUDs are not prone to misuse because you can't forget to take them (like the pill) or misuse it (like condoms). So you're protected from pregnancy 24/7 for 3 to 12 years, depending on which kind you get. Once your IUD is in place, you don't have to think about it until it expires. You can take it out whenever you choose. IUDs won't affect your fertility or make it harder to get pregnant in the future.

Manufacturers of hormonal IUDs (Mirena, Kyleena, Skyla, and Liletta) claim that they can reduce cramps and make women's periods lighter. Some people stop getting periods at all. Hormonal IUDs help treat people who suffer from severe cramps, heavy periods, and anemia.

IUD Side Effects

Some women experience adverse side effects after inserting an IUD into their vaginas. However, the side effects go away within six months once the woman's body gets used to the IUD. The adverse side effects include:

- Moderate pain upon receiving the IUD

- Cramping or backaches after getting the IUD
- Occasional spotting between periods
- More substantial bleeding and cramps

Spermicide

Spermicide is birth control that contains chemicals that stop sperm from reaching an egg. A woman puts it in her vagina before sex to prevent pregnancy by blocking the sperm from entering the cervix and getting to her egg.

Women do not need a prescription for spermicide, and most drugstores and supermarkets sell it. Spermicide packages are portable, so you can take them wherever you go.

Women can apply spermicide before sex to avoid pausing the action. Women can also use spermicide as a part of foreplay by having their partners put the spermicide in their vaginas.

Spermicide Side Effects

Spermicide may irritate a woman's sensitive genital tissues, primarily if she uses it many times in one day. The irritation may increase her risk of exposure to HIV and other STDs as the itching gives infections a pathway into her body. Also, some women experience an allergic attack after using the substance. Other side effects include the following:

- The woman's vagina or her mate's penis feels sore after using the cream.
- Spermicide could flow out of a woman's vagina.

On Birth Control Methods

- It may also taste a little funky.

Vasectomy

Vasectomy is a simple surgery. The doctor cuts or blocks the tiny tubes that carry sperm inside a man's scrotum. So sperm can't leave the man's body and cause pregnancy. The procedure is speedy, and the man can go home the same day. Also, it is about 100% effective.

A man should only get a vasectomy if he is 100% sure he does not want to get any woman pregnant for the rest of his life. Vasectomies are get-it-and-forget-it birth control, and it does not interfere with his sexual activities, such as in the heat of the moment.

Vasectomy does not screw up a man's sex appetite or alter how he has an orgasm or ejaculates. His cum will still look, feel, and taste the same after a vasectomy. A vasectomy eliminates a man's concern about pregnancy, so it can strengthen his relationship and make intimacy more enjoyable and sex more spontaneous as he and his partner focus on each other instead of birth control.

Vasectomies Side Effect

Vasectomy is a surgical deconstruction of male vas deferens (the duct through which sperm flows to the ejaculation duct). It is permanent, so a man can't change his mind later. So like all medical procedures, vasectomies have the following risks:

- Vasectomies are permanent.
- Fertility may never come back after vasectomy

- Reversing vasectomy surgery is complicated and expensive
- Reversal surgery doesn't always work

Birth Control Patch

The patch is less expensive birth control a woman wears on the skin of her belly, upper arm, butt, or back. The patch releases hormones that prevent pregnancy for three weeks. So she gets it, takes a week off, and repeats the cycle. The birth control patch is not just for birth control; The birth control patch contains hormones that make women's periods regular, lessen cramps, lighten bleeding, and protect against pelvic inflammation. The birth control patch can also reduce the following:

- Acne
- Thinning of the bone
- Breasts and ovarian cysts
- ectopic pregnancy
- endometrial and ovarian cancers
- severe ovaries, fallopian tubal, and uterus infections
- iron deficiency (anemia)
- PMS (premenstrual syndrome)

On Birth Control Methods

Patch Side Effects

The patch's adverse side effects are as follows:

- Bleeding between a woman's periods, breast tenderness, headaches, and nausea.

- Some women notice soreness on the point of patch insertion.

- Patch birth control could make a woman feel bad.

Birth Control Shot

The birth control shot, also called DMPA, contains hormones that prevent ovulation. So when there's no egg in the woman's fallopian tube, she can't get pregnant. It also makes cervical mucus thicker. When the slime on the cervix is more viscous, the sperm can't get through.

The birth control shot is convenient and easy to get. Women who hate taking a pill daily or using birth control that interrupts sex prefer it. It makes sex better for women who use it because they don't have to interrupt sex or worry about pregnancy.

Half of the women who use the shot stop getting their periods after about a year of using the birth control shot. So she doesn't worry about getting pregnant for one year. However, women who use the birth control shot complain about bleeding longer and spots between their periods. The shot helps protect women from cancer of the uterus and ectopic pregnancy. The birth control shot is reversible, so a woman can get pregnant after using it.

Although the shot does not change a woman's ability to get pregnant in the long run, it can delay it for about nine months. So, women who plan to get pregnant within the next year should seek a doctor's or nurse's advice about other birth control options.

Shot Side Effects

Some women who get the shot experience adverse side effects. "Most of these symptoms go away in about three months," the maker says. However, some women use birth control shots without any side effects. The common side effects of the birth control shot are:

- A noticeable change in the women's periods
- Substantial and longer bleeding
- Occasional spotting between periods or no periods
- Most women who use the birth control shot stop getting their period
- Nausea
- Weight gain
- Headaches
- Breast tenderness
- Loss of hair on the head or more hair on their face or body
- Depression
- Light bruising on the point of an insert of the shot

On Birth Control Methods

Birth Control Ring

The birth control ring is an affordable method a woman wears inside her vagina, where her vaginal lining absorbs the hormones. The ring is flexible and prevents pregnancy by releasing hormones into a woman's body. The NuvaRing stops sperm from meeting an egg. The birth control ring can help reduce:

- Acne
- Thinning of the bone
- Breasts and ovarian cysts
- ectopic pregnancy
- endometrial and ovarian cancers
- severe ovarian, fallopian tubes, and uterus infections
- iron deficiency (anemia)
- PMS (premenstrual syndrome)

NuvaRing Side Effects

The manufacturer claims that some women who use the ring experience annoying side effects while using NuvaRing, "but the symptoms go away after about three months." The side effects of the birth control ring include the following:

- Occasional spotting or bleeding between periods
- Sore breasts, nausea, or headaches
- Noticeable wetness of the woman's vagina

- Change of a woman's sexual desire because of the hormones in the ring.

Cervical Cap

A cervical cap is a small soft silicone cup shaped like a sailor's hat. A woman puts it deep inside her vagina to cover her cervix and stop sperm from joining her egg. The type of cervical cap available in the U.S. is called FemCap. A cervical cap works best with spermicide (cream or gel that kills sperm). A woman can put her cervical cap in place before having sex or before things get hot and heavy. Most men don't feel the cervical cap during sex. Also, knowing that your mate can't get pregnant can help you relax and enjoy sex more. Women who prefer non-hormonal birth control, or can't use birth control methods with hormones because of medical problems, find a cervical cap a good option.

With proper care, Cervical caps only need to be replaced every year. So a woman can use it many times. A nurse or doctor should check her cervical cap fitness after pregnancy.

Disadvantages of Cervical Caps

Some women have trouble inserting their cervical cap, which can take practice to get comfortable doing. The problems with the cervical cap are:

- Cervical caps could move out of place during sex if they get bumped around.

On Birth Control Methods

- Also, cervical caps don't work unless the woman uses them with spermicide. She must ensure she puts her cervical cap-plus spermicide before sex and leaves it inside her vagina for at least 6 hours after sex. If she has sex again while the Cervical cap is in her, she has to put more spermicide in her vagina. She should not leave her cervical cap in place for more than two days or 48 hours.

Diaphragm

A diaphragm is a soft silicon form of birth control that's a shallow cup shaped like a small saucer. To use it, a woman bends it in half and inserts it inside her vagina to cover her cervix.

Diaphragms are portable, reusable, and do not contain the hormone that concerns women. They start working immediately, and a woman can get pregnant as soon as she stops using them.

A woman can put her diaphragm in for up to 2 hours before having sex (that's how long the chemicals in spermicide work). Most men and their partners don't feel the diaphragm during sex. Knowing that a woman can't get pregnant while using a diaphragm can help her relax and enjoy sex more. Because of medical problems, women who prefer non-hormonal birth control or can't use hormonal birth control methods find diaphragms a good option.

Diaphragms last about two years with proper care, and a woman can use them repeatedly. It's good for a woman to have a doctor or nurse check her diaphragm's fit after a year, if she gains or loses much weight, or after being pregnant (whether or not she gave birth).

Disadvantages of Diaphragms

For a woman's diaphragm to work as well as possible, she must use it correctly every time she has vaginal sex.

- Some women have trouble inserting their diaphragm.

- Diaphragms could move out of place if the woman's mate does much thrusting.

- Diaphragms don't work unless the woman uses them with spermicide.

Fertility Awareness Method

Fertility awareness methods help a woman track her menstrual cycle and know when she is ovulating. The days near ovulation her fertile days, or the days she is fertile. So women who use FAMs avoid sex or use another type of birth control method when she is likely to get pregnant. The three FAMs that help a woman track her fertility signs, which she could use together or separately to predict when she'll ovulate, are:

- The Temperature Method: a woman takes her temperature in the morning every day before getting out of bed.

- The Cervical Mucus Method: a woman checks her cervical mucus (vaginal discharge) daily.

- The Calendar Method: a woman charts her menstrual cycle on a calendar.

On Birth Control Methods

The Standard Days Method

Standard days birth control is when a woman tracks her menstrual cycle for several months to determine if her period is always between 26 and 32 days apart. However, she could not use this method if her period was longer than 32 days or shorter than 26 days.

Once a woman establishes that her cycle is in the desired range, she could avoid vaginal sex on the 9th to 18th day, when she's likely to get pregnant or use another type of contraceptive. The benefits of fertility awareness methods are:

- They are free

- Have no side effects,

- Help you learn about your body and your fertility.

It's most effective to use all 3 of these birth control methods.

Abstinence

Abstinence is when you don't have sex—you turn away and say, "I don't like sex."

Tubal Ligation

Female sterilization, also known as tubal ligation, or "getting a woman's tubes tied," is a surgical procedure that permanently prevents pregnancy. After the doctor performs the surgery and says it's safe for the woman to have sex without birth control, she does not have to do it again. Sterilization is get-it-and-forget-it birth control.

Tubal ligation is a good option for women who prefer non-hormonal birth control due to medical problems because it does not contain hormones to prevent pregnancy. It won't cause menopause, change the woman's periods, or mess with her natural hormones. Tubal ligation does not interfere with sex. So a woman who has had tubal ligation can have passionate sex uninterrupted.

Tubal Ligation Side Effects

Tubal ligation is permanent, so the woman who gets the procedure can't change her mind later. Side effects of sterilization are:

- Getting sterilization reversed is expensive and complicated
- Sterilization reversal does not always work
- The woman's fertility may never come back.
- Rash, swelling, trouble breathing
- Fever
- Continuous pain in the woman's belly
- Abnormal discharge or odor from a woman's vagina
- Fainting spells
- Bleeding or pus at the point doctor made the incision
- Chance ectopic pregnancy
- Rare chance of sterilization reversing itself

On Birth Control Methods

Withdrawal Method

Up to this moment, the emphasis has been on convenience, not interrupting the sexual act, easiness of application, light in weight and shape, the beginning and the end of its effectiveness, and impact on women's period. However, the toxic nature of all these birth control methods and their long-term effect on the health and well-being of those who use them deserve equal attention.

Withdrawal birth control is pulling the penis out of the vagina before ejaculation because if semen (cum) gets in a woman's vagina, she could get pregnant.

So ejaculating away from a woman's vulva or vagina prevents pregnancy. So her male partner must pull his penis out of the woman's vagina before his semen comes out every time they have vaginal sex for it to work. Women use withdrawal birth control for the following reasons:

- It is free and always an option.

- There's nothing to buy

- It has no side effects

- There's nothing to put in place before sex.

Withdrawal birth control can be used by anyone, anywhere, and anytime, although it may take practice to get it right. The withdrawal method is always available if a woman forgets her regular birth control or doesn't have condoms on hand. It would help if you underlined, penciled in, or highlighted this method because that's all this book is about and the main topic of discussion in the following parts.

Disadvantages of Withdrawal

The first reason the withdrawal method fails is pulling the penis out before ejaculation (cumming). Many men plan on withdrawing and then forget or change their minds in the heat of the moment. Men have to remove their penis right around the time those pleasurable sex feelings are most intense, which many men can't do when it comes down to it.

- If a man ejaculates inside or the outer genitalia of his mate's vagina, sperm cells could swim into the vagina and cause pregnancy.

- For men who experience premature ejaculation, withdrawal birth control is not an excellent way to prevent pregnancy. Premature ejaculation is common and means you ejaculate (cum) before you're ready or realize it will happen. Especially for younger guys, it'll probably be hard to use the withdrawal method successfully.

- Withdrawal is also not the best method if you can't predict when you're going to ejaculate, are sexually inexperienced, or don't trust yourself to remove the penis at the height of sexual pleasure.

The withdrawal method requires self-control and mutual trust. It also requires a healthy relationship, where both mates are equally committed to preventing pregnancy by using the withdrawal correctly.

On Birth Control Methods

Table of Method's Percent Effectiveness

One crucial piece of information we found while researching this book which in itself eliminates any doubt as to whether or not withdrawal is among the mainstream birth control methods, is the report published by the Center for Disease Control:

In this report, the government listed all the recognized birth control methods in order of their percent effectiveness, as shown below:

Birth Control Type By Effectiveness	Percent Success	Percent Failure
Implant	99	00.05
IUD	99	00.80
Vasectomy	99	00.15
Hysterectomy	99	00.50
Injectable	94	06.00
Pill	91	09.00
Patch	91	09.00

Ring	91	09.00
Diaphragm	88	12.00
Male Condom	82	18.00
Female Condom	79	21.00
Withdrawal	78	22.00
Sponge	76	24.00
Fertility-Awareness Based	76	24.00
Spermicide	72	28.00

Withdrawal in the Media

The withdrawal birth control technique is no longer something people whisper or talk about behind closed doors. It is gaining popularity, receiving attention, and finding its well

On Birth Control Methods

overdue coverage by the media.

However, the withdrawal has not gained as much prominence as it deserves. The easiest to understand logic is that withdrawal birth control is not a product one buys from the drug store or medicine doctors prescribe. It is not a product any distributor can buy and sell in a large volume and earn millions in profit. Nobody is out there in public, promoting it or purchasing advertisements in the media to praise its effectiveness. So, it is like 'out of sight, out of mind.`

Worse still, high school sex education teachers try to frighten young people with unsubstantiated claims about the withdrawal method. Once you tell young people something is terrible, it is difficult to change their minds. Another important reason is that the withdrawal birth control method is a private behavior nobody wants to disclose, or a few want to share with their friends.

For the most part, one has to learn how to do it correctly, and it takes time, awareness, and persistence to master the act. The male partner has to earn his female partner's trust and prove that he can withdraw his penis from the vagina before the cum arrives.

There is no doubt that the media covers events with a certain tabloid overtone, which means it has to be a quantifiable failure or success to grab the media's attention. It has to be a destructive action, behavior, or incident to force the media to cover it. So we are surprised to find the media coverage of withdrawal birth control, and it is all you need to convince yourself that "withdrawal birth control" is effective. And the fears, doubts, and scare tactics the health care service providers employ to turn people against it are waning as more people discover that the practice is as effective as even the most effective birth control in the market today.

Most people denounce using scare tactics to shape public opinion and discourage people from adopting the withdrawal. However, government agencies and public health service providers often find it challenging to promote the withdrawal of the birth control method for fear that people would misuse the information. In this case, they fear people would attempt to practice withdrawal birth control without learning how to do so correctly. So it is not surprising that government agencies, public health service providers, and birth control researchers take a firm whack at the withdrawal in discussing birth control issues.

We also discovered that you couldn't discuss withdrawal within the narrow confinement of unwanted pregnancy prevention without considering other issues such as sexually transmitted diseases. And that is the central sticking point and why most researchers don't support withdrawal even when a few find it as effective as the most effective birth control, such as the condom.

One of the many pleasant surprises we encountered while researching this book was numerous articles online by the media and comments by people who read them. You can visit these websites and read the articles by entering "withdrawal birth control" in your favorite search engine.

Cases and Legal Complaints

There are legal issues associated with most birth control. However, most women love their birth control so much that they blindly think it is safe and, for various reasons, do not do due

On Birth Control Methods

diligence before using their birth control of choice.

Before using any birth control, please google birth control cases, lawsuits, and legal complaints, followed by your birth control of choice. Review the lawsuits, verify the birth control safety and the manufacturer's advertised claims, and take the appropriate precautions.

Cost of Birth Control

We reviewed the list of birth control methods, checked their prices, and found that the cheapest birth control's average annual cost, such as condoms and diaphragm, ranges from fifty to three hundred and fifty dollars. Those birth controls requiring prescription range from six hundred to eight hundred and fifty dollars. And the most expensive, including the irreversible methods such as ligation and vasectomy, vary from one thousand to six thousand dollars. However, the withdrawal method does not cost anything.

PART 3

NAKED

COMPASSION

On Smart Pullout

The most effective and safe birth control is in men's minds and their mates' giggling faces.

On Smart Pullout

Pursuit of Good Health

Never let your sense of morals prevent you from doing what is right.

~ Isaac Asimov

✱✱✱

In the last parts of this book, we referred to removing the penis from a woman's vagina before ejaculation as 'withdrawal birth control.' To some extent, men perform withdrawal instinctively without awareness and a genuine understanding of how to do it reliably and effectively. So the rest of this book provides the knowledge and awareness required to transform withdrawal birth control into "Smart Pullout" birth control by teaching men how the level of their sexual pleasure changes as sperm reaches various vital men's sex organs. And the appropriate moment to pull their penises out of the woman's vagina.

Most men practice the pullout birth control methods because they genuinely care about their mate's well-being and are concerned about the side effect of traditional birth control. Others don't like how sex feels with a condom. The task is to teach men how to pull out effectively and confidently and allow their mates to enjoy the comfort of their mate's commendable efforts.

Nobody is to blame for not pulling out effectively because, until now, unlike traditional birth control, there is no user guide for pulling out correctly. After all, who can blame someone who

Naked Compassion

takes on a task he knows little about without help or guidance? Hence Naked Compassion provides the essential guide to inspire men to adopt the technique and prevent their mates from putting toxic substances into their bodies. If practiced with inspired compassion and strict adherence to the guide, it is free, readily available, effortless, and works to perfection.

After reading this book, you'd agree that replacing "withdrawal birth control" with "smart pullout birth control" makes sense. The following points are worth remembering while thinking about sexual activity:

- Women bear a disproportionate share of the burden arising from sexual intercourse. And the least a man can do is play an active part in unwanted pregnancy prevention, not only for equity but also for recognizing and appreciating that she is the gatekeeper of life and the baby's caretaker.

- The implication here is not that men cannot be joy-givers; instead, it acknowledges all the emotional and physical burdens a woman bears after every intimate moment.

- Every baby entering this world deserves to be wanted and welcomed with joy and happiness.

- The mother deserves that fantastic heartwarming look of pleasure on her face the first time she holds her newborn. Not the look of anguish and despair because she did not want the baby.

On Smart Pullout

- Pregnancy prevention should not induce other illnesses by side effects or produce abnormal stress.

- Pregnancy prevention should be a mutual effort to strengthen the couple's relationship with the male partner playing a significant role.

The Benefits of Sex

This section contains the essential life-enhancing benefits of sex and why smart pullout is highly effective in allowing mates to harness its full benefits.

Whenever I think of the fantastic benefits of passionate sex, I wonder if every man knows the essential part good sex plays in his life, such as good health, fitness, and tranquility of mind and soul.

Sex is a very delicate topic to discuss. And undoubtedly, the most important functional aspect of human experience that everyone indulges in with a sense of giddiness and, sometimes, a conflicting sense of guarded glee and discomfort, but it represents a primary source of happiness.

Uninformed adults mention a female's insemination with a wince, virtuous hyper-sensitivity, and flawed conservative reservation. Still, the desire for sex is not different from hunger for food or thirst for water; both contribute to life's sustenance in different ways. Nevertheless, most men consider this aspect of human activities their métiers. Yet, women dismiss it with a jeer. To some extent, though, there's a large segment of men whose understanding of sex is limited to their in-out-and-repeat movement during sexual intercourse.

On the other hand, women dwell on the size and length of men's penis, unmet needs, and lack of understanding of those needs. Women know how gullible men are and are aware of the various ways to stroke their ego, so they often fake certain sexual acts and joke about it with their female friends long after the game is over—when ladies get together for chit-chat like on the View. You can't help the amusement from these enduring gender dynamics.

Men waste an unnecessary amount of energy to bring their mates to submission—something like calling out their names and dismissing their lack of immediate response as nothing but pretense. For most men who talk about sex, the only thing that matters is an orgasm—how their mate screamed aloud and called them daddy. They even suggest that it doesn't matter to a woman whether sex lasts for one, two, or three seconds—it's the joining with a man that's cherished—bull-crap.

Men's obsession with orgasm and the shame of being unable to make it happen creates their insecurity when not reassured of their prowess. Such insecurity further forces them into an abject moodiness and the wrong attitude towards their mates.

On the flip side, women torment and mock their mates for their failings, lack of knowledge of the art of lovemaking, and an elevated false sense of self-regard with glee. These feelings create women's ambivalence and knock-yourself-out attitude during sexual intercourse. When women get together, the popular topic that generates the most laughter and cheer is fake orgasms to satisfy their men's egos.

In some ways, as funny as it may seem, women think of men and their desire for sex as children around the kitchen table with a basket of cookies staring at them. They want to get as

On Smart Pullout

much as they can, get the hell out, and come back when they want some more.

Sex is a multimillion-dollar industry; the playboy magazine, the hustler magazine, the strip clubs, the pornographic stores, and now the internet pornographic sites are all designed to lure men and take advantage of their gullibility for sexual fantasies. There's even a TV show dedicated to exposing men's gullibility to seduction 'To Catch the Predator,` which they'd deny until they are in handcuff and on their way to the jail—holding cell.

For couples who are not as close and intimate as they should be, Naked Compassion could help them achieve mutual trust and closeness and enjoy a better sexual experience.

There are a few good reasons to discuss safe and enjoyable sex and how mates can accrue its benefits.

I watched TV once, and suddenly, the host interviewed a clinical psychologist whose name I'd forgotten. As the interview progressed, she began to enumerate the benefits of sex:

- "Having sex often can do more than make you feel closer to your mate—it can make you feel happier and physically healthier," she said, citing a clinical professor of obstetrics and gynecology at Columbia University. She cited other research by psychology professors from different parts of the world.

- "People who have sex at least once over two weeks were better able to handle stressful situations," she said, attributing the reason to endorphins and oxytocin, which the body releases during sex and these hormones help the brain to sense the intimacy and relax to stave off anxiety and depression. She continued to say that you don't have to climax to net the effects. However, orgasm helps you get the most significant surge of hormones; just one more reason to go for a climactic finish!

- "Hormones like endorphins and prolactin released during sexual orgasm help prime women to sleep, and a high level of prolactin accompanied by deep sleep indicates a dynamic, happy relationship."

- "Highly active sex leads to high energy rather than sleep, but slow subdued sex is indeed a sleep aid, so it's up to mates to decide what they want out of a particular session."

- "Talking about ache, pain, and anger, she suggested that good O' sex offers immense relief for pain, aches, and anger. The hormone endorphins resemble morphine, and they effectively relieve pain."

- "Some studies found that people who have sex regularly have higher levels of an antibody called immunoglobulin."

- "People who enjoyed lots of sex with their steady mates about four times a week look ten years younger than their actual age," she said. "The study concluded that having sex a few times a week causes the body to release testosterone and estrogen, that keep the body looking young and vital; estrogen does an excellent job of improving soft skin and shiny hair—the glow."

- "Aside from strengthening a woman's ticker and a good workout, she will also get some sculpting, and her abs,

On Smart Pullout

muscles in her back, butt, and thighs get a good workout as you thrust during sex," she said, citing another researcher.

Then she went on to talk about the factors that impact sex:

- "Hypo-active-sexual-desire-disorder is a condition in which people experience significantly reduced sexual desire and absence or lack of fantasy, which can lead to personal distress or no interest in sexual intercourse. She warned against confusing that condition with the issue of arousal, which can make people nervous because they feel like they can't perform."

- "Sexual aversion desire disorder is a condition that makes people feel disgusted with sex or even turned off completely." She suggested that these conditions can be psychological and medical, as well.

- "The way a child grew up and the child's experience growing up can lead to his or her adult sexual health and behavior."

- "One's social condition could lead to one or both of the above issues," she concluded.

Cultural Effects

In some cultures, people do not talk about sex. They do it and pretend it does not happen. Advanced societies have struggled to allow public utterances of sex but cringe when it's called specific names considered offensive. Individual terms are universally acceptable, although uttered in the public arena with discomfort. In many underdeveloped societies, young people marry as early as thirteen due to the culture that prohibits dating in those cultures. So all the conflicting beliefs and norms about sex make the topic of sex and the pantomimic view of people having sex on the large TV screen gossip-worthy. So we enjoy gossiping about it and watching the action in the actors' screenplay—even if we suck at it ourselves.

Some religions believe sex is sinful and should only happen for procreation—after mates are married, we know how that ends. Don't you wonder where people who cannot have children—for biological and medical reasons and others who do not want to have children belong in all these?

Changing Attitude

People's cultural background can complicate their outlook on sex, making it difficult to enjoy sex. In this case, people feel guilty or ashamed. So it is most accurate of the people in various underdeveloped countries in which sex is had only for procreation. One can only sympathize with people in these countries, knowing their conflicting emotions. Again, one can see Naked Compassion helping people gain some degree of consciousness and understanding of the importance of sex in their relationships.

Intrinsic Causes

Intrinsic causes of sexual attitude changes relate to issues arising from the relationship's state or dynamic functionality. These conditions assert themselves when things are not going smoothly. One or both mates feel unhappy due to financial issues, job-related matters, or the attitude either mate deemed

On Smart Pullout

spiteful or disrespectful. This book cannot help in such a situation except hope that the trust built from practicing the "smart pullout" would engender enough closeness and help the couple resolve their differences.

Mindset

Mindset goes to the heart of the cause of most problems in sexual relationships. For instance, men regard their mate's orgasm as a mandate rather than a source of pleasure, well-being, and other benefits discussed earlier. For this reason, they feel nervous when their mates don't express audible signs when they orgasm, forcing the female to fake it. So the male feels inadequate when he doesn't perform. Naked Compassion may help reshape mindsets when people trust each other, realize the benefits of sex, do it the right way, and engage in an enjoyable mutual activity.

Teenager's Views

Once my girlfriend engaged her son in a discussion about sex. A few minutes into the debate, he tells his mother that he knows everything about sex. So his mother said, "tell me everything you know, son."

"Maa, I'm not stupid," he said, "all I have to do is wear some rubber and stick my dick inside the vagina."

"I am glad that you are thinking of safe sex," she said, "but I don't want you to run around having sex with every girl you come across." Then she turned to me and said, "I can't believe my baby is having sex already."

"He is seventeen," I replied without offering any advice.

This passage tells you all you need to know about the status

Naked Compassion

quo, the general perception, and young people's sexual habits.

Pullout and Social Mores

Most sexually active adults consider Social mores first, as usual, before trying the pullout pregnancy prevention method, even as a test drive. Despite the pressure from these mores, Its sustainable appeal and effectiveness cannot be ignored because it is always available, costs nothing, aggravates no allergies, enhances pleasure, and has no adverse side effects.

Smart-pullout does not suffer accessibility barriers women complain about and still protects a woman's privacy, do-no-harm, and violet nobody's rights.

Mates do it for their well-being without worrying about who sees the woman going into any doctor's office, picking up items on the shelf of a drug store, or stressing over having forgotten to take some pill and putting something on before the sexual intercourse.

Perception

Perception upon which mores rely can be dangerous because it is what people hear, what they think, rumors, and false narratives—not the factual information that leads to a sensible decision. The truth is that life and death, health, and well-being, are too important to be left to perception. As you can see below, people adopt a lifestyle because it makes them feel good at a heavy price.

- At one time, cigarette smoking was cool until many smokers began to die from lung cancer.

On Smart Pullout

- Drunkenness was cool until many people began to crash their cars and die from DUI.

- Rich buttery food was once the must-have treat until it became dangerous.

- A large slab of beef used to be on the rich man's daily menu until many died of high cholesterol and heart disease, forcing them to change their eating habits.

Hard Facts

Facts do not cease to exist because they are ignored.

~ Aldous Huxley

Many people do not take the pullout birth control method seriously. Nevertheless, women who had had a bad experience with their birth control method and others who strive to live a healthy life with the minimum level of medicine or toxic substances in their bodies depend on it.

Most women who use the traditional birth control methods find the volume and scope of the information they consume from the media daunting and wonder how to make sense of what they hear before deciding what is best for them. Often fear and perception win and force people to make decisions that contradict everything in their best interest.

While researching traditional birth control, I suddenly realized that each birth control is toxic medicine in its own right. Similarly, the accuracy of the information I found is challenging to ascertain, as in our food. Some food tastes delicious or looks mouth-watering. But in reality, those food are tough to digest, and some are hard to metabolize with little or no health benefits.

Naked Compassion

Facts often collide with false narratives and win because they leave data trails along the way.

More Than Orgasm

Most of us indulge in sexual activities with only one thing in mind—to get a quick nut, turn over and go to sleep, or get up and leave. Then afterward, we brag about our self-professed expertise in lovemaking. Not that it is anybody's business who boasts about what. However, it would be better to demonstrate compassion by adopting the "smart pullout" technique instead of focusing on the performance that often falls short of expectations.

There is no doubt that the common theme in most discussions about sex is "orgasm" Most people experience it or have experienced it. Very often, it's the end goal for the participants. Most men like to know they did great, so their mates fake it to stroke their egos. I call it orgasmic fascination.

Beyond orgasm, the sexual pleasure and ecstasy that delight in seductive, erotic acts, and feminine beauty, men should pay appreciable attention to females' well-being in all matters relating to sex and pregnancy.

Enjoying a Bit of Each Other

It is not hard to understand why sex does not feel good when you have sex wearing a condom unless you're one of those people who delight in intense visceral sensations. And, your only goal is physical exercise, or you love to be a woman's dildo—sharing nothing.

On Smart Pullout

The body contains millions of sensitive tissues (neuro sensors) that communicate with the brain back and forth through the neuro transceivers. I'm trying to say that the feelings we get from sex when the male and female organs are in flesh-to-flesh contact are utterly different from those we get with prophylactic.

Common sense tells us that when two bodies immerse in the precum, they experience some feel-good sensation that produces an enjoyable feeling. It causes the brain to make chemicals and fluids to maintain our hormones or immune systems. Anyways, this is a job best left to researchers.

You can test this assertion by knocking yourself out with masturbation and seeing if you get the same deep sleep, feeling on top of the world, or glowing the following day from having passionate sex the excellent O' fashion way.

Undoubtedly, the "smart pullout" allows you to enjoy sexual intercourse and reap its benefits. So this is what you get from having gratifying sex without a condom:

- You'd experience a significant temporary reduction of the accumulated stress you'd been having.

- Muscular fitness from enjoyable exercise—stretching and pumping.

- Your body creates hormones that keep you feeling happy.

- The good mood and on-top-of-the-world feeling you get after good sex translate into focus and allow you to do your job better or elevate your sense of pride.

- It strengthens your immune system, which fights infections and keeps you healthy.

Naked Compassion

Validation and Effectiveness

When the government states in a report that the pullout, which is so derided and maligned in public, is seventy-eight percent effective, the chance is that its effectiveness is much higher—say 88 to 90 percent. The point worth mentioning is that if people use the pullout with such high percent effectiveness, common sense suggests that the number would be in the nineties if people learned how to pull out confidently.

Pullout may not work for every couple. However, the question is, why is it so?

Unlike other birth control products, the pullout is not something you take, put on, rub yourself with, sit back, and wait for it to work. It is a practice that culminates in a standard of living; hence, it works excellently well for those who master the act.

Some women don't hesitate to deride the pullout; some say they don't know anybody who does the pullout, as we call it, because they have had enough sex education courses and know damn well that it doesn't do the job.

If you are like many people who have had enough sex Ed and don't believe that you need more information or lessons on the pullout, you can skip to the "Worksheet" section, cover the answer section, and answer the quizzes before checking out the answers. If you get all the answers correct, "Congratulations," you are on your way to mastering the act of the pullout. But if you did not get all the answers correct, you can continue to read and learn how to pull out successfully.

Another phrase the critics use to describe the pullout birth

On Smart Pullout

control is that it is something left to "hope and prayer" if you feel that way, you need to read this book to the end and reconsider.

As to whether or not the pullout is authentic birth control, there are three ways to evaluate the claim:

- The mere fact that the pullout is among the government-listed and recognized birth control methods makes it a legitimate birth control method.

- The intense adverse reaction the pullout gets when researchers and journalists publish their findings illustrates its value that drug makers don't want you to know.

- The increasing number of people who switched their birth control method of choice and turned to the pullout yearly demonstrates how acceptable it has become.

Most of the points and concerns often raised in the discussion of the pullout birth control are genuine. Because they reflect how the average person who has not learned the act would feel about anything they are about to do for the first time without a user's guide.

As men learn how to pull out successfully and confidently and adopt STI prevention described later, ultimately, pullout will become self-validating for the following reasons:

- It is safe, free of charge, and highly effective

- It is readily available

- It guarantees you complete privacy

- It lets you reap the full benefit of sexual intercourse.

PART 4

NAKED

COMPASSION

On STI Prevention

There is no greater agony than knowing you could have prevented the pain you feel.

On STI Prevention

Safe Sex

I feel so safe knowing that I have sex every time with the same woman I knew was healthy when we began our relationship.

✱✱✱

To the extent that fear, self-preservation, and common sense allow, we can assume that not every horny adult carries sexually transmitted diseases, so the question becomes:

How can you protect yourself from being infected?

The typical answer or the knee-jerk response is always "use the condom" without considering how it makes people feel. Sure, for people who like to have sex the first time they meet the person they are attracted to,

The obvious answer is to wear a condom! However, suppose you are dating to start a relationship. In that case, the reliable approach is spelled out in this passage because it allows the mates to enjoy all the good feelings and vital benefits of passionate sex.

This method of preventing sexually transmitted infections relies on the virtues of fidelity and loyalty between mates who love and depend only on each other for their sexual needs. I am aware that some readers will jump all over this concept and describe it as unattainable;

However, if you're in an inspired relationship and like what you see, enjoy how you feel, and love what you crave, everything that makes fidelity and loyalty unattainable becomes trivial, like a crack on the road you can easily step over.

I must concede; that finding a mate who inspires fidelity and loyalty is not easy. But it is possible if you search for one and do your due diligence patiently.

So how do you start?

First, let me say that it helps to start dating in high school or college, learn different aspects of human social behavior, and wear a condom if you have sex during this freelancing period. Because it is at this early stage in life, people become aware of those human attributes that light up their emotional fire, put it off, or keep it flaming. Also, maybe give their cerebral selves the chance to form the basis for making the right relationship choice later in their lives.

Here is how to go about it:

The most commonsense way to start is to do an initial blood test—both of you. Please review it to ensure that both of you enter the relationship with a clean bill of health. By doing this, you are applying the principles of "Trust and Verify." Then maintain subsequent blood tests and keep records you can review periodically to ascertain your good health.

Reasonable Option

Regardless of how you feel about sex, it fulfills vital natural needs—happiness, joy, good health, and tranquility of mind and soul apart from baby-making needs. The "smart pullout" offers

On STI Prevention

the reader a reasonable option that protects human sexual pleasure, prevents unwanted pregnancy, protects against sexually transmitted infections naturally without pills, cuts, and stitches, or artificial or toxic substances inside the sacred and holy part of a woman's body.

To learn more about Smart Pullout, refer to the section titled Resources, and sign up for online private training at half the price with the purchase of this book.

Important Steps

- First, make sure you've done due diligence after meeting somebody you like. Ensure that your feelings have staying power by convincing yourself that your mate's favorable attributes are far higher than the unfavorable ones.

- Talk about smart pullout and stress the importance of fidelity and loyalty in preventing sexually transmitted infections.

- Finally, take a blood test periodically, share, and discuss the result to mutually convince you and your mate that you are starting your relationship with a clean bill of health.

If you have sex with only one healthy person, you eliminate the possibility of contracting sexually transmitted infections and guard against sexually transmitted diseases.

WARNING: Combining sexually transmitted infection prevention and unwanted pregnancy prevention is the most attractive feature of smart pullout birth control. For additional information, turn to the section titled "Resources."

PART 5

NAKED
COMPASSION

On Building Confidence

I don't mind being the first, but I feel more confident knowing that people have done and succeeded at what I want to do/

Naked Compassion

Fear Doubt and Endorsement

***

One of the Center for Disease Control reports we reviewed put the pullout second among the most tried birth control forms among the teenagers surveyed. Still, the report gave the pullout thumbs-down, which is not surprising because of apparent sneering by the government agencies and corporate institutions at anything that promotes the pullout and fails to suggest that it is worth studying to help people use it efficiently and correctly. Instead, they use scare tactics to discourage women from seriously considering the pullout; they label the thought ill-conceived, irresponsible, and, worse yet, call the women who use the pullout ignorant. So in this book, I try to show that it could be a well-conceived, responsible and informed exercise for people who learned to do it correctly.

The government's net effect on the pullout instills fear and doubt in women and compels them to turn their backs on the safest form of birth control that would allow them to live with the least amount of toxic or cancer-causing agents in their bodies.

Surprisingly, women themselves are the most vocal critics of the pullout. They stigmatize each other for using the pullout, and their religious beliefs fuel the fire. Still, women who rely on the pullout as their only birth control method provide a different narrative that refutes the notion that the pullout users are lazy, uninformed, or ignorant. They are intelligent, educated, critical thinkers and fact-based decision-makers.

On Building Confidence

However, this narrative's bright side is that more women realize that the pullout is a healthy alternative to any other birth control. The earlier reports show that they endorse its use in large numbers.

For the six years I lived with my girlfriend, Doreen, she engaged her friends in their group discussions about birth control issues. In most cases I'd listen and take notes, but in some cases she'd ask me to talk about the pullout while she served as a credible witness of whatever I had to say about it. When Doreen and I first met, she would not entertain any discussion about the pullout or suggestion of its use because she learned in her high school sex education class that the pullout is a non-starter if a girl doesn't want to get pregnant. But after I proved that I could do it efficiently, she became an advocate of the pullout and tried to convince her friends to try it.

So everywhere we lived, Chicago IL, Evanston IL, Waukegan IL, Minneapolis MN, Minnetonka MN, St Luis Park, MN, and Plymouth MN, she talked about the pullout. I remember one occasion Doreen's best friend, Sharleen, ran out of the pill and asked Doreen for some. She was shocked when Doreen told her that she had stopped using any form of birth control. She screamed at Doreen, cussed her out, and called her stupid for doing what the sex education teachers said didn't work in high school. Then her other friend, Tamika, seemed personally offended and yelled, "you can't possibly trust this man to know what he is doing."

Several women among the well over a hundred we met had tried the pullout, and many depended on it as their reliable birth control method. However, they disclaim it as risky openly for fear of what their friends would think of them. Some women who had never had a baby because they used the pullout feared they might be infertile if it was unreliable. Below is some of what the women Doreen talked to about the pullout:

In Their Own Words

I used the pullout for one full year without any problem. The best part is whether you are with someone or alone; you don't worry about getting pregnant or putting some shit in your body.

—Yvonne, Chicago, IL

I get mad when I hear the so-called smart people talking down the pullout. My boyfriend and I relied upon it for 12 years. We were in a long-term, monogamous relationship, and I enjoyed sex every time without worrying about blowing up, getting pregnant, or catching any birth control side-effect.

—Charity, Chicago, IL

I asked my gynecologist what she thought of the pullout, and I was like, wow, when she said, "Several of the medical professionals I included are sympathetic to the pullout use but afraid to admit it publicly." There's a stigma among many educators and medical providers."

—Kelly, Chicago, IL

The whole thing is a scam. There's a perception that young people should use condoms every time they have sex, and saying anything positive about the pullout will discourage that. Corporations and their army of lobbyists supported by the FDA want us to keep putting dirt in our bodies, and they don't care if

On Building Confidence

we catch cancer doing that. They make tons of money off women who use their product; nobody makes a dime promoting the pullout. They can't say anything positive about the pullout, even the possibility of using it successfully, which means there's more going on than STI concerns.

—Margaretta, Chicago, IL

It is not the government's attitude towards the pullout that worries me but the pervasive belief among women that drives them to reject men's capability to pull their penises out of women's vaginas when they are ready to cum. The direct result is a social environment that regards men as lust-filled animals who can't control themselves when they bump and grind with their women. So this trend of thought pushes women to think that the pullout is unreliable and engenders mistrust between a man and his mate. The prevalent mistrust between partners is often the major problem with the pullout birth control method. Some people say it gives a man far too much control; others say the pullout gives him the responsibility he cannot handle. And the whole idea is complicated by the notion that men won't be able to sense when it is the right time to pull out, or they won't even try because cumming inside a woman feels better.

—John, Chicago, IL

You guys are missing the critical point in this discussion. It is all about making money. No one profits from telling people how to pull themselves out of a woman's body when they cum. No one makes money doing it; there is nothing to sell or buy here. So the corporations do not give a damn. You cannot get funding telling people to do it, and you cannot find funding to test it and present the result for FDA approval. We are all

Naked Compassion

screwed, but I must say, despite all the skepticism, it is a healthy alternative to all other birth control methods out there, and we just have to continue to do our thing as best as we can.

—William, Skokie, IL

I have been in a long-term relationship with Sam for 13 years; breaking news, we are getting married this summer; we use the pullout method, and I have not gotten pregnant in all those 13 years. You have to work on it together and make it the real thing. It is the best birth control because it allows you to enjoy each other.

—Maggie, Waukegan, IL

That's all crap. It does not work. When I was in college and out on a one-night simple, quick grab, I did not have my condom with me, so I let this guy who said he could pull out try it, and I got pregnant with my son. This shit is a joke; I should have known better.

—Candice, Skokie, IL

I conceived once when a condom broke inside my vagina and a second time while I was on the pill. So I abandoned the so-called conventional birth control and turned to the pullout. Mark and I have used it for twenty-four years without adding to the two kids we already had. You can make the pullout work if you care about each other and work together. Another thing, it makes your relationship stronger.

—Cassy, Evanston, IL

On Building Confidence

Do you girls know that no birth control is foolproof? I got pregnant while on the pill and IUD, so I am reluctant to return to other birth control except for the pullout.

—Marybeth, St Louis Park, MN

I feel ashamed to discuss the topic of the pullout method; it is risky. It is what men say to women to get a piece of ass; it does not work. I tried it once in high school and got pregnant because my boyfriend did not like wearing condoms, and I wasn't on birth control.

—Denise, St Louis Park, MN

My husband and I used the FAM with the pullout for years because I didn't want to be on any birth control, and my husband hated the condom. It worked ninety-nine percent of the time. The other one percent was when he cried so loud, and I laughed and got distracted instead of helping him pull out.

—Kristen, Skokie, IL

I have to tell you all; women are crazy. We complain men don't care when we cramp. We complain men can't give us orgasms. We complain all men want a quick nut and nothing about how we feel. Women complain that men don't care whether we get pregnant or not, and for the few who care and want to try to help, we still can't trust them. What do we want from them? And why can't we give them credit for trying? Maybe you all should become lesbians that way; we can talk about other things instead of how untrustworthy men are. It is ludicrous to hear people make a blanket assertion that the pullout doesn't work. Hello! It is not a product and certainly not a medicine. It is what people do by and for themselves.

Naked Compassion

Therefore, it is as effective as you make it. Ken and I rely on it, and I help him pull out every time we have sex for six years.

—Liz, Waukegan, IL

I started dating my fiancé when I was fifteen and sixteen. We did not have sex for a year because I was afraid my dad would kill me if I got pregnant, so we waited until he got his apartment, then we researched birth control, and the side effects of birth control scared the Jesus out of me. We found that some hurt the mood and contain crazy hormones that cause women's health issues. The manufacturers have settled cases out of court and claimed no responsibility for getting women sick. So my fiancé and I began to use the pullout with FAM. At first, it was like, OK, if it doesn't work out, we will get married before anybody knows I am pregnant. It was some work at the beginning for my confessional girls until my fiancé, Ben, got very good at it. We both enjoy making love so much that Ben would do anything to make me comfortable when cramping. The pullout is all I know about birth control, and I have no complaints.

—Eve, Minnetonka, MN

I used the heat calendar and the pullout method because I wouldn't say I liked any birth control, and my husband hated to wear a condom. It worked very well except once when I got pregnant.

—Lady, Minnetonka, MN

I don't know about you girls; I never enjoyed sex until I got

On Building Confidence

on the pullout. Karl and I are beaming with happiness regarding satisfaction in our sex lives. I am glad that my body is doing its thing naturally and that I don't have to worry about the birth control side effects. I credit the pullout for getting us to where marriage is on the horizon, and we will have children when we decide to do so. When we feel it is risky to use the pullout or near my ovulation period, we give sex a break or do it in conjunction with the FAM; there's far less stress doing it that way. I give Jim lots of credit because he has practiced this art for years and knows the right time to pull out. I hear some women use the pullout method in conjunction with condoms instead of the pullout method, but I think that defeats the purpose because you can't enjoy sex with the condom. I feel a stronger bond with Jim because the trust is there, which is essential. After all, it would be best if you trusted your partner to pull out in time, and he trusted you to be honest about where you are in your cycle. Another thing is communication; it has to be there, like other aspects of your relationship.

—Gladice, Plymouth, MN

I haven't met anybody on the pullout you ladies are yapping about; I am in a monogamous relationship, and I don't use it. Many people have had enough sex education courses to know that it doesn't work most of the time, and too many sex education classes have condemned it as risky.

—Nancy, Brockton, MA

When I told my co-worker I was using it. She said, "you are using the "pull and cross your finger" method. She thinks she is smart, but I tell her she is simply ignorant.

—MaryAnn, Dorchester, MA

Naked Compassion

Honestly, every woman has tried the pullout in their relationships. That's just the conventional contraception method that everybody tries at one point or another in their sex lives. I like it because it is a natural feeling that is much better than using a condom. I don't blame girls who use the pill and pull out because we've been scared to death with horror stories of unwanted pregnancies caused by the pullout mishap. Many women use the pullout as their sole birth control when they have sex with somebody they trust doesn't have STD (trust is the key). Sometimes it makes no sense to rely on this method alone. Still, when you consider other birth control methods' horrible side effects, especially what the hormones do to your body, you are left with no other sensible option.

—Caroline, Brookline, MA

The bottom line is that you have to be strategic and realistic at the same time. It will fail at one point or another, just like every other birth control method. My sister was married for ten years and on the pullout before her first child. She relied on the pill from junior high to her 20s, and then she went off the Pill when she married. She did not think it was a good idea to hop back on the pill, mainly because she gained a lot of weight while on the birth control pill, so she went on the pullout. After her first child, she did not worry about getting pregnant and relied solely on the pullout for over twenty years. It was a massive success until she got pregnant at 46 in December. My sister called it 'Kirk's Christmas surprise gift`. It was a big surprise for the entire family, but considering no birth control method is foolproof, it shouldn't have been such a shock! And being

On Building Confidence

married to a great guy made the whole thing less of an issue.
—Elizabeth, Cambridge, MA

How It All Began For Me

One Saturday afternoon in 1967, I was seventeen and enjoying the record Unforgettable by Nat King Cole when I heard a knock on my door. I ushered the visitor—the girl I met a few weeks earlier- and left the door open while the curtain gave us the necessary privacy. We sat on the floor by the stereo set and played a few classical records—by Jim Reeves, Brook Benton, Elvis Presley, and Duke Ellington. As the afternoon waned and evening rolled in, we decided to spend intimate moments. I loaded the record This Magic Moment by the Drifters in my stereo set and jumped back into the bed. Immediately, we found ourselves in a state of sexual ecstasy— naked and wrapped around each other. My hand wandered over her beautiful face as we listened to the music. I felt bumps and rashes on her face, and I went around them softly, disregarding them as a typical pimple.

Now squeezed by the natural urge and the fear of entering into a world I have only been barely in once—not quite sure if I made it all the way. The desire prevailed, the music continued to play, and I surrendered. A few minutes after my girlfriend lets me into this new world of hers, I felt a pinch inside. It was Oh-my-God!-moment for me because a cousin of mine (She and I were born on the same day—a few minutes apart) had warned me once that girls are nothing but trouble.

So not knowing what she meant by "girls are nothing but trouble," I became an instant believer thinking that the problem she had warned me about was real. So I pulled away from her, thinking, "yes, girls are worse than trouble; they are dangerous. Something in them bites a man's penis during sexual intercourse."

After realizing my reason for pulling away and jumping up, she grabbed my hands and asked me to sit down. Then she told me all about the object in her body. She explained that her mother had put that copper loop in there because she would get pregnant if she had sex without it. I must confess to absolute ignorance on the matter of sex and pregnancy.

Yes, I was seventeen—old enough to know, but I did not because nobody talked about sex when I was growing up; that adults had sex for pleasure was a myth, and as for pregnancy, it was only supposed to happen after people are married. So she began to explain in vivid graphic terms what would happen if we had sex without that protection—pregnancy that would have changed the course of our lives.

"I feel sore in there and bleed sometimes," she said. "I wish my mother had not put that copper inside my body."

Then she took my hand, let me feel the rashes on her face again, and said, "I started getting these pimples and rashes on my face after my mother made me wear that copper." For good reasons, and because I had used copper in electrical wiring, I opined that inserting copper in a girl's body was harsh, abnormal, and cruel.

I was overwhelmed by the pure, innocent sense of empathy and compassion. I poured my indignant heart out at the doctor and my girlfriend's mother for putting anything in that sacred place—inside my beautiful girlfriend's body. So we cuddled as my mind reached inwards as deep as it could, searching for the

On Building Confidence

alternative to that copper-insert she called intrauterine device.

As the evening rolled along and darkness crept in, everything suddenly changed when my girlfriend decided to cook dinner before leaving. While cooking, she cut vegetables, added condiments to the soup as my mother used to, and let me stir in the seasoning.

Though I cannot say how I would have felt if we had had sex, we enjoyed the time we spent in the kitchen together so much that it took my mind off that IUD disaster. Later that evening, after escorting her to the bus stop, I returned to my apartment, and something profound happened. Most men my age would have derided and left her. But I did the opposite.

I decided I would be the kind of man my father was to my mother in every way—her trusted partner and care for her in unique ways. So when she visited again, we discussed how to have sex without hitting that copper insert inside her body.

For a while, we did. Then I began to think of what I would do to convince my girlfriend to remove the copper in her body. Then I ran into a problem. I was a complete novice about everything regarding sexual activities. Then I remembered what my father told me once, even though my girlfriend and I were not married yet nor started a steady friendship:

Man's primary responsibility is to protect, defend, and care for his wife when she needs it.

The next time she visited, I told her I would like to pull my penis out of her vagina when I reached the climax so she wouldn't have to wear that copper insert. However, I wasn't sure how I would accomplish my goal, so I began thinking of something acceptable to us both. "You are completely out of your mind," she said. "No man can pull that thing out without dropping some in there."

"We would never know unless we try," I said.

No matter how much I tried, I failed to believe that my girlfriend was safe wearing IUD. I grew up with my cousin and heard people chastise her for not closing her legs or sitting upright when we sat down and played some children's games together; I had listened to her friends curse her out for wrestling with me like a boy. As time went on, I watched her worry about her period because she could not go to certain places with me while on her period. Regrettably, the culture forbade girls from entering certain areas in the village while they were on their menstrual period. So I wondered why she should bear such an unfair burden for what she did not bring about.

Knowing that my girlfriend is wearing a copper inserted in her body's most sacred part to prevent her from unwanted pregnancy bothered me. Therefore, for the second time, a sense of righteous indignation against society forced me to conclude that:

Unlike boys, every girl comes into this world with an unfair social burden.

So I pledged never to allow my girlfriends to bear those burdens alone. For that reason, I decided immediately to take over the responsibility of preventing her from getting pregnant and let her have the peace of mind I believed she deserved. So I began to learn how to have sex with her without putting a drop of semen inside her. However, the problem was that I was

On Building Confidence

attempting to do something I did not fully understand.

Nevertheless, I continued with what I called "Shared Reasoned Action." I began to think of ways—not well thought out due to a lack of understanding of what I was attempting to do. Like most people, neither my girlfriend nor I knew anything about the organs that make up male and female reproductive systems. So we had to rely on instinct, feelings, tone, and tenor of our interactive voices. Without talking or uttering the word intrauterine device again, we began playing around between her laps to test if I could pull my penis out before the cum erupted.

Honestly, my first go at it was an absolute disaster that dragged laughter and giggles out of my girlfriend. Yes, she laughed and jeered at me because I failed woefully to predict precisely when the cum was about to erupt, even though the signs were right there.

That jeer and laughter are exactly the reactions everybody gets when they begin to practice the "smart pullout." You should expect—dragging funny-relationship-strengthening teasing responses out of your mate when you start to practice the "smart pullout" birth control. In my case, it became a weapon with which she shot at me occasionally when I was in a bad mood. So I cleaned myself up, determined to be mindful of the changing levels of my sexual pleasure—sperm-induced feelings, and predict its arrival better next time. The next time we practiced our new act, I did better and better during each successive lovemaking until I mastered the act.

By mastering the act, I mean—we got to a point where I would scream, "I am cumming" remove my penis out of her vagina, and we would watch the semen erupt. Six months later, I made a believer out of her, and the next thing I noticed, she had removed the intrauterine device, and she did not have to worry

Naked Compassion

about getting pregnant for as long as she had sex with me.

Yes, we started with that intrauterine device in her body until I perfected the act, which I demonstrated persistently—time after time before she took the copper out. We had sex without the fear of unwanted pregnancy while we were dating. Then we lived together and had sex every night except the four days of every month, during which nature wouldn't allow us to have sex. Eventually, we got married and had three children—we had planned.

Considering my novice of the reproductive systems at the time and complete ignorance about the birth control methods, an act of "Naked Compassion" sprung from my deep sense of love, caring, and empathy. Since then, I can proudly say that I have had quite a few girlfriends—six to be exact over my sixty-some years of active sexual life and functional dynamic relationships without getting one of my girlfriends pregnant.

Condom Aversion

Tremont Street is a major road linking Boston with Cambridge, Massachusetts. Just across and opposite the famous Boston Commons is McDonald's restaurant, where young students from various high schools, colleges, and universities within the city work to make a few dollars to pay their tuition fees and have fun. I owned a Toyota Corolla car, and I enjoyed clubbing and movie-going. I worked the closing hours while others worked rotating shifts. So I worked with every employee as their schedules switched through my working hours.

The first afternoon I worked with one of the female employees, Aisha West, it became apparent that working at that

On Building Confidence

shop would be fun as we set off sparks flying everywhere.

Right out of the gate, she ordered me to mop the floor as if she was the manager, so I said no. Then she called me hot-head. From that moment, we bickered every time she tried to dominate me. Usually, our drama ended with her telling me, "you are too stubborn to listen to anybody." And I'd reply, "Only anyone named Aisha West."

Aisha was the same height as me and stunning in many ways. Her shining black skin seemed always moisturized and captivated boys around her. Aisha was fascinated by my accent and mimicked almost everything I said. Still, she introduced me to her sister as her boyfriend, notwithstanding the hell she was putting me through at work.

I would drop her off after work, come home, and lay awake all night, missing her as if we had been away forever, even though I had just left her for minutes. Luckily, I did not have a telephone in my apartment, so I did not burn my tuition money talking to her on the phone.

I did not care about movies that much, but when she dragged me to the movie, she would do sweet, friendly things that would work me up to an ecstatic frenzy, and I would come home wishing the film had never ended. The next day at work, she would tell me she did not sleep well because she kept thinking about our last time together.

We had fallen in love, and we knew it.

Aisha's father worked for the city of Boston, and her mother worked at the Filene's store at the Chestnut Hill Mall. She told her mother I was paying my way through college, and her mother thought it was fantastic. One evening, Aisha said, "In

Naked Compassion

our neighborhood, holding a job is kind of cool, and doing so to pay your way through college, well, that is something to brag about," which she did all the time.

One evening, while Aisha and I were cooking dinner, I told her I needed a second job. "Why do you need a second job?" She asked. Then I said, "I don't have enough money to pay my tuition before school starts." Instead of reasoning with me, Aisha said, "I think you would have saved enough if you were not running around with girls." So I asked her, "who exactly are the other girls? You were the only girl I was running around with the last time I checked. Do you want us to break up?" Aisha punched me in the stomach and said, "no, stupid. I mean Lynne and Eleanor."

Suddenly, her mother entered the house and greeted us, "how are you guys doing?"

"Your son-in-law needs a weekend job."

"Why does he need a weekend job?" Mrs. West asked.

"He needs a few more dollars to pay his tuition fees before school starts," Aisha replied.

"Ok, daughter," her mother replied, "why don't you help your husband find a weekend job?"

She reached into her bag and gave us a newspaper to search through the part-time job advertisements section. We did just that and found a job opening in her company; cashier and housekeeping positions.

A few days later, she gave me gas money and told us to come to Chestnut Hill mall—a southside suburban town of Boston, for an interview. We attended the job interview and got hired. We worked on Saturdays and Sundays. Aisha worked in

On Building Confidence

customer service, and I kept the isles clean and threw totes, wrapping materials and cardboard away all day.

We still worked at McDonald's Monday through Friday, forcing and bumping into each other as always when we worked together. It was a routine for us. We stayed apart most of the time at the mall except when her department needed my service. We ate at the cafeteria together during our thirty-minute lunch break, stepped on each other's toes, and snatched each other's carton of apple juice—a habit we always enjoyed.

One day, while delivering a few wrapping paper boxes to Mrs. West's counter, she asked how the tuition money was progressing. "I have enough to pay my tuition fees," I said.

"That's great," she said encouragingly. As a back-to-school present, Mr. West gave us fifty dollars to go out and celebrate our hard work. So we went out that evening, not knowing a surprise lurking in the wind, and our friendship was about to die a sudden death. We had dinner at McDonald's with our friends at work that evening. Then we went to the movie and watched "The Kung Fu Fight."

Lost in the thrills of the moment and everything else Aisha did in the darkness, the three-hour movie seemed like a ten-minute slide show. When the film ended, we left the theater singing:

"Everybody was Kung Fu fighting" along the way home in the car. We got close to Aisha's house, and then she asked me to make a "U" turn. So I did. At this moment, our relationship was on a high-altitude automatic cruise mode. In some ways, that's what it felt like to me. "Where are we heading now?" I asked,

"To your apartment," she replied. I must confess to finding myself in an elevated state of anxiety—afraid of what would happen next and how it would affect the illusory image of me she had mistakenly created in her mind.

Suddenly, I found myself in a state of euphoria, as that inner enemy—wicked testosterone drove my desire to fever-pitch. Worse yet, I could not anticipate what would happen to my affection for Aisha.

The feeling I had from having Aisha slip a condom on me stepped in the way and ripped everything apart.

We got to my apartment, staged a mock Kung Fu fight, and took a bath. She brought a flat-pack out as we played in bed, ripped it open, and slipped it on me. It was my first experience—an introduction to the condom. So I did not know what to expect, nor was I opposed to using it. I could have said no and told Aisha about the pullout I had been practicing all my life till then, but I did not. Like all virgin acts, the first one broke because of something I'm not bold enough to say but rather leave to your imagination. Nevertheless, she brought out another pack and proceeded to put it on.

Minutes after Aisha put the second condom on me, my feelings began to recede like the ebb of a tide, and my body recoiled. "What's wrong," she asked,

"I don't know."

Suddenly, nothing was left of my desire for sex, and, disappointingly, my interest in Aisha dipped to a freezing point.

It was the most negative transformational event I had ever experienced. "What's wrong with you," Aisha asked again "everybody uses this shit. You should have told me you don't want to make love to me."

On Building Confidence

"I've been yearning for this moment," I replied, "I don't know what happened. I've never felt like this before."

At that moment, it was apparent that things would never be the same again. I felt as though that was the end of our friendship. So I gave Aisha a ride home, feeling ashamed. And wondering what was wrong with me. If everybody uses condoms, as Aisha said, why then was it a disaster for me? It wasn't merely a condom mishap. I must be averse to a condom, I concluded.

After dropping Aisha off, I went home and slept without thinking of her—for the first time. When I went to work the following day, I saw a different person, and her beauty lost its allure in my eyes. It seemed as though I'd lost the most precious part of me; I felt like dying.

For weeks, I faked my affection and love for Aisha. I became a false me—a fake person yearning for escape from awkward moments whenever we were together, and when we were apart, she became non-existence. I struggled to understand why my feelings, love, and affection for Aisha crumbled to what I then called benign neglect—an unexpected result of having a condom slipped on me.

Everything has gone wrong, and it's nobody's fault. Imagine that!

In many ways, that is how I felt when I lost my affection for Aisha. I felt crushed, dead inside, as my feelings and fantasies twirled around in what seemed like an emotional storm.

Acting cold towards Aisha as I did, although involuntarily, was the worst behavior I'd ever indulged in, even though she did nothing to warrant it. However, as with every young person in my situation, the moment's significance was beyond my grasp—

can you blame me? So I tried a few more times, and at every instance, my body grew colder and recoiled further until Aisha concluded that I did not love her enough to want to make love to her. "All you have to do is say so," she said. Just imagine the feeling.

But she was wrong. I can't imagine anybody not wanting to make love to a girl like Aisha. No! It was not a matter of love, like, or desire because I had been looking forward to that moment, yearning for her touch to uncontrollably restlessness whenever she touched me. Before the first condom snapped, my vital sex-ready indicator was jumping out of me. I knew it was not a matter of want; it could not have been a lack of desire. I had been dying to make love to her and euphoric just before she put that condom on me

I am condom averse! I will never allow anybody to put a condom on me again.

This anecdote is significant for two apparent reasons. First, women do not know how men feel while making love with condoms. Second, there are no books on how most birth control methods affect relationships. Instead, the prevailing view is that everybody who is not making love for the sole purpose of having a baby should use condoms to protect against pregnancy and sexually transmitted infections.

However, this chain of thought seems to consider sex a visceral physical exercise ignoring human sensitivities and the overall benefits of sex. It also appears to regard everybody as a disease carrier from whom we should protect ourselves, ignoring

On Building Confidence

some other sensible alternative such as pullout and sticking to having sex only with that one healthy person from whom we derive our sexual pleasure.

So here we are, unsure of the most reasonable way of having sex, enjoying it, and protecting against pregnancy and sexually transmitted infections. Sure, Naked Compassion contains a sensible method to prevent unwanted pregnancy, guard against sexually transmitted diseases, and ensure that people enjoy sex and its benefits—when it's well done! And that is what this book offers.

Uncomfortable Truth

One day, we were sitting in my brother-in-law's living room in Union, New Jersey—just yapping about the current events. Suddenly one lady began to berate young girls for having babies before marriage. The topic gathered momentum as other people echoed the same sentiment. I wondered aloud— saying, "this situation would have been different if those young couples had learned and practiced the "smart pullout" pregnancy prevention method, which I have been practicing since the age of seventeen."

I sat there and listened to the guests and their wives attack the young girls for having babies and me for saying that boys could play a significant role in preventing unwanted babies. So I questioned why they don't exhibit the same outrage for the boys who got the girls pregnant. One lady who seemed very confident in her opinion said, "boys do not have babies girls do." To balance the argument, I asked, "would any girl have a baby without a boy putting sperm in her?"

I broadened the issue by asking, "if boys refuse to wear condoms and girls refuse to use birth control, how could they

Naked Compassion

prevent the pregnancy?" The wise lady raised her voice and yelled, "Any girl who refuses to use birth control is stupid." Sensing that the argument was getting personal, I reminded them that after one marriage and about seven relationships, most of which lasted for over six years, I never got one lady pregnant except for the three daughters I had with my wife. So I decided to write this book to reach a larger audience and encourage boys to practice the smart pullout if they can't wear a condom.

Doreen's Story

I woke up one Saturday morning in the intensive care unit of a hospital on the west side of Chicago; my children—a boy and a girl had been in the hospital for two weeks for smoke inhalation from the fire that burned my apartment down while I was at work. On that day, my babysitter had left my children alone in the apartment and went out to cash her check. Then my son torched the apartment by turning on the gas stove.

Although the doctor had discharged my children that morning, my son was still in a daze with a continuous non-blinking stare and would not respond to anything around him, so the doctor concluded that he had suffered brain damage. I had dropped my kids off at my sister's house and stopped at my mother's to lay down for a few hours of sleep before breakfast.

When I woke up, my mother sent me to the neighborhood store to buy bread and a pack of eggs for breakfast, and that's when I met one young man. After hearing about the kids and that I was literarily homeless, he took us in. He took care of my kids like they were his and applied every lesson he learned in psychology classes to get my kids to regain a healthy life.

On Building Confidence

Now six months had passed, two since the doctor declared that my kids were back to normal again and a few weeks since my man had enrolled the kids in kindergarten and daycare. Chuks has cared for us without making any sexual moves even though his body parts seem to be running out of patience, as they'd let me know when I make contact with them. At this moment, I knew I was with a decent man who would not allow himself to come off as caring for us for sex. So I decided it was time to take the initiative and let him know I appreciated him.

One evening, I cooked a nice dinner and set the scene with candlelight, the sweet aroma of burning incense, and a long hot relaxing bubble bath. At dinner, Chuks was all smiles and seemed thrilled with the scenery and delighted with my sense of romance. But when we went to bed and things got heated, and the mood was perfect, I brought out a pack of Trojan condoms, then his mood changed. He put the package back in my hand and asked me to put it away.

Instead of having sex, we cuddled while I listened to how he lost a beautiful girlfriend once when she slid a condom on his penis, and his body and feelings for the girl died suddenly. It was less than an inspiring story. So I felt sad.

He told me about the pullout birth control method he had practiced since he was seventeen.

"That's bull crap; you can't do that," I replied.

So my libido raged on, and Chuks stuck to his guns until one day, he suggested that we try it on one of my safe days. Sensing I was coming round to agreeing, he said, "If I scream to signal the arrival of the cum, just push me away from you." So we did, and he surprised me because when he was about to ejaculate, he screamed, "I'm cumming" and pulled away, and then we watched the cum rush out. We lived together for six years and had sex every night except for those crampy days; I did not take any pills because he pulled that shit out every time. And I did not get pregnant even though I would typically get pregnant once I forgot to take my tablet, and for the period we lived together, I did not worry about getting pregnant. Then I became the most vocal advocate of the pullout.

Sheron's Story

It has been three months since Chuks and I met, yet the topic of sex did not come up even though we went out on dates regularly. It was the first time a man did not ask me for sex after going out that long, so I began to suspect that he might be gay. However, he had talked about his ex-wife and children. So one night out, I made my move and put a pack of a condom on the pillow. His mood changed, so he chose not to have sex rather than wear that stupid jacket, as he put it.

So we went back and forth about not wearing a condom. I told Mr. Chucks that I could not have a baby due to a narrow pelvic problem. Still, he would not give in, so I gave him the benefit of the doubt; after telling me that he had practiced the pullout since the age of seventeen, he suggested we start during my safe days. He also told me to push him away from me when he said, "I am cumming,"

So we had sex the way he liked—without wearing a condom, and as he told me just before he ejaculated, he screamed, "I'm cumming," and pulled away. He made a believer out of me because he pulled his penis out of me way before the cum rushed out. From that night until I moved south, we had sex without fear of getting pregnant.

On Building Confidence

But We Were Careful

One summer day in 1987, I came home from work while my girlfriend, Ernestine, was cooking. And her friends, Candice and her boyfriend Larry, and Kimberly and her boyfriend Smith were in the dining room chatting loudly about going to the club, getting drunk, and having sex afterward.

As always, I took my shower and joined Ernestine in the kitchen. She looked at me with discomfort, knowing some news was about to break. "Are you OK?" I inquired.

"Why do you ask?" She inquired back.

"You look visibly uncomfortable," I replied.

Suddenly, Candice broke the news, "I am pregnant by accident." So there was dead silence for a while, then Kimberly screamed, "are you stupid or what? I told you to make Larry wear a condom." Smith tells Kim to shut up, saying, "Nobody can make me wear a condom. I hate that stupid thing."

Emotions flared up, and an intense argument ensued, with everybody raising their voices and occasionally spewing cursing at each other. They went back and forth on birth control pills and quickly agreed it was a bad idea. They turned to IUDs and gave up the idea. As they went round and round in a circle, they seemed to return to the condom as their preferred birth control method, but Larry would not buy the idea, and neither would Smith. So, Kim lashed out at the men for being selfish, saying, "What we get every time we ask men to wear a condom is, no, I am not wearing that shit. They don't care; they are selfish."

At this instant, Ernestine and I served dinner and sat down to eat with our guests—some with angry faces looking away from others. Then Ernestine wanted to know if Candice did what she told her to do. "Yes, I did, but Larry was too stupid to know when he was cumming," Candice replied. Knowing how much I hate to discuss our private matters with her friends, Ernestine turned to me and said: "baby, I am sorry; I told Candice how you pull your shit out every time you are about to cum. I have to help these girls."

Despite the angry look on my face, Ernestine begs me to help Candice, Kimberly, and their boyfriends so they won't have any more unwanted babies they cannot afford to raise. For a moment, I thought Ernestine was wrong to tell her friends what we do in the privacy of our bedroom. Then I realized that women love to brag about their mates, especially when he does what they describe as—´ the right thing.` So I discussed the mechanics of the smart pullout with Larry, Smith, and their girlfriends.

"How do I know the cum is about to come out?" Larry asked.

"How do you feel when you are about to cum?" I asked.

"I feel overwhelmed by the ecstasy of the moment—"it's like something is sucking me into that shit, you know what I mean."

"Yeah, man, like you are helpless," Smith agrees.

So I told them that the overwhelming pleasure they described is the moment of ejaculation, and all that's left is for the cum to flow out of the penis; hence they must pull out immediately after they start feeling that way.

What You Should Know

The "smart pullout" pregnancy prevention technique is unique for the following reasons:

On Building Confidence

- It requires valuable knowledge of the principle known as sperm flow and position awareness (SFPA), which helps couples master the practice.

- It requires a thorough understanding of why sexual pleasure changes during sexual intercourse.

- It works without introducing any medicine or toxic substances into the female body.

- It costs nothing and causes no side effects.

Lovemaking often produces elevated sensitivity of the human reproductive nervous system. So the concept of sperm flow and position awareness (SFPA) explains sperm production, how it travels, its pathways, and how the male sexual pleasure changes as sperm arrive at various vital sex organs.

Important Questions and Answers

To adequately feel confident adopting the smart pullout, here are important questions we have to ask and their answers.

1. How do you measure the pullout's effectiveness?

You can measure the pullout effectiveness in different ways. The two that come to mind are how a statistician calculates it and how a sensible non-statistician would. A statistician would collect a hundred thousand couples who practice the "smart pullout" pregnancy prevention technique. After seven years, he'd count the number of couples who got pregnant or had children during the experiment; he would count those who did not and compute their percentages.

He could also introduce a control group of another hundred thousand couples and ask the sample universe to practice the "smart pullout" pregnancy prevention technique and the control group to go about their business as usual. Then after the experimental period, he would compare the number of couples in both groups who got pregnant and publish their percentages.

However, these approaches are flawed because they would most likely ignore the factors that affect pullout effectiveness.

The effectiveness of the "smart pullout" pregnancy prevention technique should be measured correctly to achieve a reliable result. First, take a sample group of any size who do not use condoms or withdrawal methods and compute the number of children had during the sample period, say, seven years. Then let the same group learn and apply the smart pullout for the same sample period and compute the number of children with and without the pullout.

This approach would eliminate several variables, such as medical, biological, frequency, and participants' fertility.

2. How does the smart pullout promote happiness?

Generally speaking, sex is vital for healthy living as clean water, clean air, and healthy food. Skin-to-skin sexual intercourse allows the brain to create hormones that promote a good mood and happiness. This concept makes smart pullout the

On Building Confidence

most attractive alternative to traditional birth control. Healthy sex should not be confused with sexually transmitted infection prevention which this book addresses separately.

3. Who benefits from this knowledge?

Everybody benefits from the "smart pullout." But it is not that simple for many reasons. People who do not have vaginal sex may not benefit from this practice since they do not drop sperm in the vagina in the first place, while anybody who engages in penis-vagina sexual intercourse will.

4. How would it help save marriages on the verge of collapse?

Marriage, by all accounts, suffers the same faith as love—both are fragile. Without a material and objective cooling system, it always tends to heat up to a melting point. The emotional needs of the couple do not always align. Their health needs are not always in sync. The pressure from daily activities is not generally the same. Their childbearing needs—the number of children and ways of achieving it may differ because unwanted pregnancy prevention is always the female's burden. Also, how her husband reacts to her cyclic monthly period lingers in her mind, driving the marriage's fragility to a breaking point every time a simple misunderstanding occurs. The smart pullout can help couples build the trust and closeness they need to overcome their differences.

5. How could it promote fidelity and prevent sexually transmitted infections?

Trust takes time to build and a long time to lose completely—all things being equal. When you practice smart pullout pregnancy prevention, you demonstrate a certain level of compassion and consideration that helps you and your spouse look forward to the future. Another unique feature of the "smart pullout" is the funny little behavior it brings out each time couples have sex. Such actions make the couple jeer and laugh at each other and often start conversations when they find it difficult. So since sex is a continuous activity, as is any other behavior, both reinforce each other and keep the relationship going.

6. How long will it take for the couple to master this practice?

Adopting the "smart pullout" is personal, so how long it takes to master the technique depends on the individual's determination and effort. However, three months should be plenty enough.

7. How much will it cost each month or year?

The "smart pullout" does not cost anything. It depends on the knowledge acquired from this book and the effort to understand the technique.

8. What is the side effect?

Side effects often connote something risky, disadvantageous, or medically harmful. The "smart pullout" does not have an adverse side effect. Instead, it has positive side effects, such as the desire for more frequent sex.

On Building Confidence

9. How does it help lovers to reap the full benefits of sex?

Sex has to be a flesh-to-flesh activity for the couple to enjoy its full benefits discussed earlier, so you'd be reaping all of its benefits rather than give up any benefit of sex.

Something To Talk About

The ability to initiate a conversation without thinking about what to say can be good if it is receptive or comforts the person listening. It can also be harmful if it is distasteful or generates anger. In some ways, relationships and marriage are moments where emotions' fragility is always a concern. Specific minor incidents occur, feelings flare up, and suddenly mates stop talking to each other.

Have you ever sat in a restaurant and watched a couple sitting together staring straight ahead, looking at space, and hoping the appetizer arrives in time to save the day? If they're lucky, the waiter or waitress comes along and serves the appetizer, then the couple jumps on it and munches away, still unable to look at or talk to each other.

Now you wonder what coming out for dinner is all about in the first place. The couple wanted to go out because one mate demanded it in most cases. In other instances, they mutually decided to go out as a part of their routine relationship-strengthening activities. I call this phenomenon "conversation impairment deficiency syndrome." In most cases, it does not necessarily indicate a significant problem in the relationship. Still, it highlights the need to develop conversational skills and engage in interactive activities at home and outside. And in bed as well.

Naked Compassion

Sometimes, starting a conversation is the easy part. The hard part is finding a funny teaser to arouse the other mate's interest. Generally, teasers or humor related to the mate's behavior during intimate moments works very well.

If you learn the "smart pullout" and practice it correctly, you'd find it a powerful antidote for this conversation impairment deficiency syndrome.

I must confess to being a chronic sufferer of this God-awful affliction. I've been slapped, pinched, and beaten up with a pillow because my mate could not yank a word out of me. When angry or offended, I tend to recoil and retrench into my inner shell for fear of saying something I might regret later. It's just a bad habit with nothing to do with my relationship's health or strength; it is a somewhat unconscious realization that words hurt. If you are like me, do not worry.

Here's the good news. By practicing the "smart pullout," you and your mate will build powerful teasers in your toolbox to get you talking again in moments of anger or moodiness.

Here is the tool and how it works

One night, after completing work on my book cover and going to bed, my girlfriend and I began to have a mutually satisfying lovemaking session. Then as I signaled the crescendo, pulled away, and spoke in Latin, French, or some other language or dialect I'd never heard of before, she lay on her stomach looking at me, jeering, teasing, and laughing. "Look at you, cry, baby," she said.

"Shut up," I replied, "you scream, call God, and talk funny too."

On Building Confidence

I was not talking to her for some minor offense before that moment, but after that explosive finale and the accompanying teasing and counter teasing, we began to talk and laugh again. This teasing and counter teasing is not the first, second, or even third incident of either of us not talking, only to have the funny things that happened during our sexual activity intervene and restore normalcy.

Here's another incident I will never forget. One evening, we went out for dinner at the Red Lobster restaurant, I had things on my mind, so I was not talking or even paying attention to what was happening. Suddenly my girlfriend stepped on my toes and asked me, "What's on your mind? Is it about pushing you to the floor last night?"

"No, it is not," I said, "I am thinking of that phone call last night."

"I know; it's quite unlike you," she said, "I think she got the message."

Then we began to talk about that phone call and how I engaged the caller. That's the tool, and that's how it works.

Here is how it helps to achieve a long-term relationship

There is no other situation where the pullout is more helpful than marriage. Mates are more likely than not to lay their guards down and take the longevity of their friendship for granted—the ultimate irony of the goal achieved. Most people measure their marriage by what they give, receive, or intend to get out of the relationship or rely on their legal rights for their actions.

So all the ideals they nursed, cherished, and hoped for become illusory or utterly unimportant. In some instances, revelations about the past come to light afterward and bear heavily on the marriage. Friends and relatives often creep into the marriage with devastating influence—a wicked hatchet that destroys the relationship.

But when mates feel safe and secure with each other and convinced that either is fully committed to the other's well-being, the last thing they think about is the termination of that union.

Also, when a man plays an active role in pregnancy and sexually transmitted infection prevention and helps his mate have the peace of mind to share her love and enjoy her femininity as she chooses, he makes the relationship last.

Avoiding Child Support Woes

Often lost in unwanted pregnancy discussions are young people and their ambivalence towards condom use. It is hard to believe anything will change the trend of unwanted childbirth until young people embrace a birth control method that allows them to enjoy sex—as they fantasize and prevent pregnancy.

The "smart pullout" birth control provides young people—who will never entertain the thought of wearing condoms the needed choice of having sex the way they like without making babies—they are not ready to raise. To appreciate young people's mindset regarding sex and unwanted pregnancy, you need to find the TV channels that feature shows like Jerry Springer, Steve Wilkos, and the Maury Povich Show, and watch the shows with an open mind.

By open mind, I mean without judging or condemning anybody—based on your point of view. These shows might come across as reality or freak shows the first time you watch

On Building Confidence

them. The truth is that they are typical shows that represent a part of us we'd rather pretend does not exist. For me, it was the day I walked down to the civil courthouse to take care of my parking violation fine. Then I saw tens of Jane Does vs. John Does, each disputing who the baby's father is, questioning the justice in seeking child support payment against them, and resisting restriction order.

I watched the above TV shows a few times and was astounded to find what seemed like young people were always full of their gripes and squawks over babies they had helped bring into the world and then realized that they couldn't afford to raise the baby. I do not mean to suggest that these programs do not have entertainment values—sure, they do, gripes or not. The entertainment part comes when the young couple begins to argue. It goes like this: "The baby looks like you," the girl would say, "look at her nose, ears, or eyes."

"My nose, eyes, or ears do not look like that," the boy would counter. "they look like your ex-boyfriend." This argument continues as the girl tries to prove that the boy is the baby's father, and the boy tries to convince her that he is not. Then the boy would come at the girl with what he considers to be irrefutable or ironclad evidence; "many times you said that you were going out with your friends, but my sister saw you entering your ex's house."

Also, to defend herself, the girl would say, "I told you to put on a condom, but you said no."

Then I would yell at the TV, "you should think about the "smart pullout.""

The host interrupts the argument and asks the girl why she didn't just leave the boy alone if he can't have sex without wearing a condom. "Because I love him," the girl would reply.

Naked Compassion

The I-can't-believe-this (ICBT) moment arrives when the host pulls out the DNA result with the following pronouncement:
"John Doe, you are the father." In some cases and
"John Doe, you are not the father." in others. One of the parties sprints off the stage as the crowd gasps. So the child support woes become the boy's reality—if he is the father. However, if he is not the father, the girl sobs and sprints off the stage, and that episode ends with the crowd booing. The booing, in this instance, is not about the baby. It is disapproval of the girl for having sex without a condom and with more than one boy

Child support is one way the government has tried to discourage young people from having children they have no business having in the first place, and the truth is that it hasn't worked, nor will it ever. In countless instances, boys have dropped out of school and taken on a job to comply with the court-imposed child support order. And there are other instances when the boy falls out of school entirely and refuses to work because every penny he makes goes to child support payments.

There are instances where both parties stay in school, take part-time jobs, and raise the child with their families help, but that is not common. In reality, young people want to have sex to get a nut without the thought of pregnancy or having a baby until the baby arrives, and they face child support or early marriage that will not last. So this book provides young people with the essential knowledge they need to have sex without the nightmare of paying child support, dropping out of school, which will ruin their lives, or raising an unwanted baby they cannot afford.

PART 6

NAKED
COMPASSION

On The Underlying Concept

*It is hard enough to remember my opinions without also
remembering my reasons for them!*

~ Friedrich Nietzsche

Naked Compassion

Sperm Flow and Position Awareness

I am not a teacher but an awakener.

~ *Robert Frost*

✳✳✳

Smart pullout relies on the fundamental concept of sperm flow and position awareness (SFPA). It explains how sperm flows through the male reproductive pipeline and how sexual pleasure changes as sperm reaches vital sex organs. You must talk seriously with your mate about this fantastic approach to preventing unwanted pregnancy. Adopting it would prevent pills, medicine, and toxic substances from entering your woman's body and enable her to enjoy a healthier life.

Because withdrawal birth control is what people do instinctively, whereas Smart Pullout birth control relies on knowledge and awareness of how our bodies function during sexual intercourse, we replaced withdrawal with "smart pullout."

To some extent, Naked Compassion aims to explain the mechanics of the pullout, take the mystery out of it, and educate men to apply it with confidence.

A good understanding of SFPA is the key to pulling out at the right time.

On The Underlying Concept

Most adult men have sex, get their nuts, and believe they know everything about sex because they produce sperm. Naked Compassion encourages them to go a bit further and make it worry-free.

One of the birth-control methods we covered in part 1 is the withdrawal method. We learned that it is the safest, available all the time, and costs nothing but only 73 percent effective, although the actual percentage may be much higher.

The principle of sperm flow and position awareness is the knowledge men need to make pullout 100 percent effective. The pullout is 100 percent effective for me, so I believe it could be for other men who are inspired by compassion and commitment to their girlfriend's well-being right from the start.

Getting Started

You, Will, Need Naked Compassion if you have decided to learn the "smart pullout" technique and prevent the pregnancy you do not want. People ask me many questions about the "smart pullout" pregnancy prevention technique, but the most frequently asked questions are these three:

1. How can you tell when the cum is ready to erupt?

The level of pleasure and the intensity of the sensitive tissues and membranes differ at various points along the sperm pathway. So the sensation and sexual pleasure you feel when the semen enters the urogenital diaphragm is spectacularly overwhelming, letting you know that you are about to ejaculate.

2. Where do you get the power and determination to get yourself out of your girlfriend's body before the sperm erupts?

The overriding reason for adopting the "smart pullout" birth control is compassion and the desire to prevent unwanted pregnancy without loading up the female's body with toxic substances. The eagerness to pull your penis out of your mate's vagina comes naturally from your feelings and your appreciation of her natural attributes. And the energy emanates from a man's happiness when expressing his caring and dedication to his mate's well-being. Also, knowing her reproductive system is free of toxic substances fuels a man's energy to pull out. When you set your mind on helping your girlfriend avoid unwanted pregnancy, every time both of you make love removing yourself from her body becomes a way of life. This worthwhile habit sustains the determination to pull out. However, regardless of your noble intentions, it takes effort and determination.

3. How can you tell the sperm did not drop inside the vagina or on the vulva?

The answer to this last question is a practical matter. One obvious way I rely on is to remove the penis at the onset of the overwhelming pleasure—a few seconds before the eruption and watch the sperm gush out.

If the sperm starts to flow while you are withdrawing your penis, the second but less convincing way is to let your mate stick her finger inside her vagina and decide if the wetness is due to some sperm dropped inside it or her precum wetness.

On The Underlying Concept

For the most part, I rely on the first method of clearly removing the penis from the vagina seconds before the cum eruption and verifying that the sperm started to gush out after the penis was out of the vagina. Although the goal is to achieve certainty, plan B is the answer when in doubt.

Ejaculation Delay Exercise

People often go out all night, all day, and to parties, then on their way home, they feel the urge to use the bathroom. The bladder does not wait for you to get inside your house; it does not wait for you to take off your clothes and get to the bathroom; it is entirely up to you to delay the pee from rushing out.

Most people twist their legs, move around, or dance awkwardly until the pee pushes through to the urethra, where nothing stops it from coming out. You strengthen your pelvic floor muscles by performing all these acts, allowing you to hold off your urination until you unzip your pant and aim your urinary outlet at the toilet bowl.

Another form of the same exercise is to contract your pelvic floor muscles, stop urinating midstream, and release the pee. Performing the pelvic contraction exercise enables you to get used to delaying ejaculation until you have fully pulled your penis out of your mate's vagina. Practicing ejaculation delay exercise while masturbating will also help you master the pullout technique.

You May Need More Help

The worst people say about the "smart pullout" birth control is, "it is difficult to do." Sure, this feeling comes from the fear of failure. Most people would not attempt to swim in deep water for fear of drowning, but once they learn to swim, they become eager to drive to the beach, dive right into the ocean, and enjoy the fun. Yes, every valuable act tends to be difficult initially, especially when the act requires focus, determination, and exactingness without allowance, deviation, or indulgence, as in this case. Research has shown that even for people who adopt the pullout birth control method without a thorough understanding of how the reproductive system works and lack determination and passion, the technique is still as high as over seventy-eight percent effective.

That means over seven out of ten people find this method effective—they succeed in preventing unwanted pregnancy. So imagine what the number would be if everybody practiced it correctly. I mean each mate participating in the exercise to make it successful consistently.

So, first, you must have a long discussion with your mate. It would help if you were not afraid to engage and compare it with the best traditional birth control. Argue rigorously, discuss everything about the practice, pros and cons, and the part each of you must play to pull out successfully, and then reach a mutual decision.

If you decide that the "smart pullout" is suitable for both of you and that you love the idea of preserving your woman's body, then help is possible. Suppose you would like your woman's body to function like nature intended without drugs or toxic substances. Furthermore, if you need help preventing unwanted pregnancy without cuts, stitches, and prophylactic, you need to scroll down to the section titled 'Resources' for further information.

On The Underlying Concept

Pitching The Smart Pullout

There are a few ways to bring up the "smart pullout" topic, and each depends on the circumstance under which the matter comes up. In every instance, you have to apply your best communication skills. The way you pitch this thing will likely expose how much you care about your mate and the extent to which you respect and sympathize with what she goes through daily to protect herself from the unwanted pregnancy nightmare. And make sure that both of you continue to have fun making love without the scare of unintended pregnancy. Caution, one thing you should not do is pitch it like a car salesperson and ask your mate to take a test drive, or like a character in a TV commercial and tell your mate, "just do it." The matter is too emotional to be taken lightly. The following are a few moments when the discussion of the "smart pullout" seems appropriate:

Spontaneous Moments

One instance is when either mate does not want sex, and the other mate wants to do it. Another instance is when the lady is horny or decides that her mate deserves intimacy beyond the night outing and takes the initiative. She invites her mate to her house—if they live apart or follow her mate's home. She would likely pull a condom—a pack of "Trojan" out of her purse and ask the guy to put it on or try to slip it on her mate.

Another moment is when both mates are lying in bed; she is reading a novel or texting a friend, and he is watching sports with none of them quite interested in what the other is doing, or maybe on rare occasions when both of them are viewing the same program on the TV. Suddenly, she starts to take off her mate's pajamas. The pajamas come off, and then she takes her

Naked Compassion

nightgown off and gives him a pack of "Trojan" condoms to put on or start to put the condom on herself. Now let's assume this is your moment. So what is the right thing to do in a spontaneous situation like this?

Maybe, you should consider what I have done in similar situations that made a whole lot of difference in how my reaction strengthened our relationships:

It would be best if you did not say a word—at least not yet; pull her close, very close, and closer, hold her tightly and kiss her. And then go to sleep. She may try to push or pull away from you. Please don't let go of her but if you do, let her go gently.

There are two things to keep in mind. You have just committed one of the worst offenses a man can engage in a relationship. I mean resisting his mate's advance when she takes the initiative. You may have to go far away from her to have breakfast the following day because she will not cook or eat with you.

However, don't worry, "every cloud has a silver lining" in fact, what you have done is let her know that your feeling for her goes beyond sexual pleasure—that you are a man indeed, and she'd let you know that when it is all said and done.

The following approach is what I do in typical situations when my mate and I have dated long enough (three months in most cases) and decided to take it to the next step. By that, I mean when I have asked her out, treated her to dinner at her favorite restaurants, given her flowers, taken her to movies and clubs, and proven that I am romantic—indeed her kind of man.

Then I'd make a formal request for meaningful discussion

On The Underlying Concept

at dinner, which is the best time I discuss important matters with my mates. We'd cook our favorite meal together and have dinner with a glass of wine for her and a glass of cranberry juice for me because I don't drink alcohol.

During the dinner, I'd discuss the matter of birth control, my concern for her health, and my condom aversion. If you have had experiences when condom use destroyed your affection for your girlfriend, this is the time and how you start.

Beg for her indulgence, and tell her how your story relates to condom use. Tell her your story and emphasize how much you loved the girl once, how long you dated, and how the condom ruined it.

Talk about the fun things you did on dates, places you went, events you attended, and how much fun you had clubbing. Speak to how much you yearned, craved to make love to her, and even bought the "lambskin condom" yourself the night you decided it was time for some loving. Then end the story with the anticlimax, meaning how you felt when you put a condom on.

In my experience, I was euphoric, excited, and longing to make love to my girlfriend, Aisha until she slipped a condom on my penis. Then, my feelings for her began to recede slowly until my fully erect body part shrunk, and I lost my desire for sex. It is not a feeling you forget or overcome.

So this girl, with whom I was once in love and both of us could not keep our hands off each other, became so unattractive that I could not look at her, and her voice made me feel some irritation. Although I cannot say that I hated her after that moment, I can honestly say that my once love for her turned to cold and benign neglect—a terrible feeling between love and hate.

That's what happened to me. Now it is up to you to tell your

Naked Compassion

story passionately so your girlfriend would understand how you became a condom averse. Then talk about the "smart pullout" and give her Naked Compassion—If she doesn't have a copy already. Finally, conclude this part of the discussion by letting her know that you'd have another round of conversation on birth control after she finishes reading the book. Please don't ask for her opinion—not yet!

In the next round of discussion, let her know that you have researched birth control and are concerned about the pills, inserts, and toxic substances women put into their bodies. Talk about the adverse side effects (the extent to which women do not wholly know) of all the birth control methods. Tell her how genuinely you worry about the possibility of her getting sick from any birth control method. Also, let her know about the principles laid out in the Naked Compassion.

Let her know that you are aware that everybody worries about contracting sexually transmitted diseases, and women, in particular, worry about their mates cheating on them. Then, talk about the STI prevention aspect of the "smart pullout" birth control and how it will strengthen your relationship and eliminate those fears.

Finally, let her know that what excites you the most is that you'd be avoiding toxic substances from getting into her body. Commit to taking the online course together to learn more about the pullout, which will help you master the practice and feel comfortable starting.

This last statement is the most crucial part of the discussion. Reach out, hold your girlfriend's hands, and ask, "What do you think." Don't say anything! Her answer will likely be, "let me

On The Underlying Concept

think about it." Your response should be simple; "Thank you, baby, for listening to me. Please let me know when you are ready to finish this discussion." Why are you ending the discussion this way? The answer is "to delineate this discussion from your everyday talks and how you usually communicate. So, do not bring up sex or birth control issues until she brings them up herself.

However, be prepared for her response. The temptation is to argue with her. You must not argue with her. Instead, listen carefully to her because how you feel about condoms is trivial compared to her fears of getting pregnant. If you genuinely care about her, you must state passionately and repeatedly, "I suggest this because I care about you." If she asks you questions, answer the questions honestly. If the questions are tricky to explain, say, "let me think about it."

Consistency is Key

You know your testimony is strong when your roots are so deep that other people's storms will never knock you over.

~ Shannon L. Alder

When I began to practice withdrawal birth control, I was seventeen, naïve, and ignorant of anything relating to sex. Premarital sex was forbidden and subjected the offender's family to shame and ridicule. Young people endured the urge for sex, fearing doing so would get their girlfriends pregnant even as their sexual hormones raged on and drove them insane.

Moreover, we did not have sex education in schools, so nobody thought sex was pristine, life-enhancing, and feel-good-act; boys and girls should know about, enjoy, and learn how to perform without causing pregnancy. However, this does not dismiss the possibility of unmarried people doing it with concrete family shame avoidance schemes.

So we languished in ignorance and misapprehension about everything relating to sex and pregnancy. We deceived ourselves into believing that pregnancy was an act of God that occurred when a man and a woman were alone in bed or in the darkness. So we avoided being with girls in bed and night until after graduating from high school or college. Living alone, we experience overwhelming sexual desire as our hormones rage on like wildfire. My turn came at the age of seventeen when I met my girlfriend.

As I alluded to in the section "How It All Began For Me," I thought about the pullout. I imagined doing it, and I did it to help my girlfriend deal with the side effect of IUDs. I also knew consistency was key. So I persisted in learning how to pull my penis out of her before ejaculation every time.

Unlike most young adult men, I started my sex life by helping my girlfriend avoid the nightmare of unwanted pregnancy. It began as an act of compassion and grew into a way of life—something I did every time we had sex. For that reason, we had sex as often as either of us needed a nut, then we lived together for four years, doing it a few rounds each time and daily except for four days of every month nature gave us a break, and she did not get pregnant.

After we married and decided to have children, I stopped pulling out. Then she got pregnant almost immediately. After our first child, we resumed our pullout pregnancy prevention practice, and she did not get pregnant again until we decided to

On The Underlying Concept

have another child. After the second child, we continued our pregnancy preventive measures, and she did not get pregnant for five years. Then soon after we decided to have our last child, she got pregnant again. So we had our third and final child.

That's not all. After divorcing my wife, I met a young lady who told me she was as fertile as a rabbit, so we dated cautiously for a few months, and then I told her about the pullout. As you would have imagined, she said that I was crazy. Also, she added, "I don't believe in the fairytale." However, I convinced her that it is effective as a condom. I did a blood test to alleviate her fears of sexually transmitted infections and persuaded her to do the same.

Consequently, we had sex as often as we needed a nut without worrying about getting pregnant. In short, I had become adept at the practice and vigilantly aware of how the changing sensitivities of my nervous system during sex cause changes in the level of my sexual pleasure.

A few weeks after we broke up, I ran into her and noticed she had gained weight. Unaware she had met another man and gotten pregnant, I joked, "I like your new plump look."

"I forgot that not every man knows about the pullout we practiced together," she told me. "So I got pregnant the first time I had sex with Keith."

Another appropriate anecdote is in the section titled 'Doreen's Story.' After high school, she got pregnant and had her first child—a boy while on the pill. Then she had her second child—a girl eighteen months later while her boyfriend was using the condom, and as a result, she was thinking of ligation when we met. However, she had not made up her mind. "What other reliable alternatives are there?" She kept asking herself.

Because she had had disappointing experiences using the

Naked Compassion

pill and condom, she was searching for another alternative. I knew I needed to convince her and prove that I could pull out before the cum. That means pulling out convincingly and watching the onset of the cum eruption.

Six months had now passed from the day we first met. Although the man under my underwear had become jumpy and restless—hitting every part of her—it came into contact with all night, I could not initiate the discussion about sex. The circumstances that brought us together were such that I could not even think of bringing up the topic of sex at that moment.

A fire had burned down Doreen's apartment building, and her children—one boy and one girl had been receiving treatment in the hospital intensive care unit for smoke inhalation. Coincidentally, her two babies had just been discharged from the hospital the day we met. I felt I was just another Good Samaritan.

Nevertheless, Doreen talked about sex occasionally and from the expression on her face. I could tell that she was drowning in a sea of ambivalence. Her resentment that condoms could not protect her from unwanted pregnancy was apparent. And the hormonal pressure to get some nut was evident from how her hands would wander around and grab a part of me that I am sure you can guess what she was grabbing. Still, we held back until her children recovered well enough to start kindergarten and daycare.

When she felt comfortable enough and decided to have sex, she would not do it without a prophylactic, and I would not do it with a stupid jacket. Instead, I told her about the pullout that she dismissed immediately and laughed off, saying, "You could do

On The Underlying Concept

better than that." So we had a stand-off for a few weeks, then she decided to give me the benefit of the doubt, and she warned,

"If I get pregnant, I will not have an abortion; I already have these two I never wanted."

More important than the pullout was how she expressed her appreciation of the practice and how it led to our lasting mutual trust.

No! She did not get pregnant for the seven years we lived together.

Finally, I moved to New Jersey in 1998 and met another young lady. She had been married, divorced, and had three daughters. Her youngest daughter was thirteen months old. While we were dating, she told me horror stories of her battle with birth control side effects and made it clear that she did not want another baby. Even after I told her about the pullout pregnancy prevention technique, she dismissed it as artifice—something a man says to get some ass.

"You cannot convince me that it is impossible," she said.

So then, three months later, after hearing how my one-time girlfriend, Aisha, killed my sexual desire by slipping the condom on me, she gave in, and the fun began. It's like Déjà vu. So after demonstrating my ability to pull out ahead of the cum out-rush, we grew close and became inseparable.

Unsurprisingly, It did not take long before she confessed to enjoying sex more than before and credited the "smart pullout" for her new passion. Whenever I think about her confessional, I wish every woman would experience the joy of worry-free sex the way they had always fantasized. By this, I mean expressing their femininity and enjoying sexual pleasure without the fear of getting pregnant.

In essence, the Smart Pullout engenders trust and

Naked Compassion

appreciation, making trips to stores such as "Victoria Secret" or "Marcy's" to pick up a few items like lingerie or body works and sensual perfumes like Red Door or Dark Obsession, a habit like going to the grocery store.

Also, you will most likely enjoy the comfort of lying in each other's arms and going to sleep, and when you have some energy left, joke and tell each other stories. Like the crazy things Dad said you should not do, you snuck out and did them anyway, or the people Mom cautioned you to stay away from, but you snuck out and dated them and spent nights in the city.

My satisfaction with "smart pullout" lies in knowing that I did not make a baby I did not want. My exes cherish the relationship we had and still love to see me.

The ultimate goal of the "smart pullout" is to get people who are genuinely in love to the point where they can have only the babies they want and build mutual trust that leads to a lasting relationship.

PART 7

NAKED
COMPASSION

On Reproductive Organs

Any fool can know. The point is to understand.

~ Albert Einstein

On Reproductive Organs

Male Reproductive Organs

*It's never alluring; it does not fascinate; it's not nice-looking
enough to dress up or gossip-worthy to get anybody interested.
"Oh! Come on, the balls?" they never look great.*

✳✳✳

Understanding men's reproductive system is essential to
mastering the "smart pullout." This part contains the names and
descriptions of the individual organs that constitute the male
reproductive system.

Scrotum

The scrotum is a combination of skin and muscles, and it is
under the penis. Also, it contains a pair of testicles. The muscles
allow it to maintain a comfortable distance between the testicles
and other parts of the body and support sperm creation.

Testicles

The pair of testicles reside inside side by side in a pouch
and connect to the abdomen. They contain a complex structure
of small containers called lobes. Each lobe has a section of
seminiferous tubes, lining with epithelial cells responsible for
sperm and testosterone creation.

Epididymis

The epididymis is a long thin tube tightly wound into a

Naked Compassion

mass that lines the top edges of the testicles' back. It stores the sperm produced in the testicles, keeps it there to mature, and moves it into the male sperm pipeline.

Vas Deferens

The vas deferens is the male sperm pipeline. It carries mobile sperm from the epididymis to the ejaculatory tube through the abdominal cavity.

Ampulla

The ampulla is behind the bladder and the rectum. And it is the broader part of the vas deferens that connects to the ejaculatory duct.

Ejaculatory Duct

The ejaculatory tube is the portion of the vas deferens that connects the prostate and the seminal vesicle. It is the final part of the vas deferens where a large amount of the fluid and chemicals from the seminal vesicle and the prostate combine to convert the sperm to semen.

Seminal Vesicles

Two seminal vesicles are at the back of the urinary bladder and the front of the rectum. The two small lumpy glands connect to the ejaculatory tube and produce the chemicals that convert sperm to semen that can swim upstream inside the vagina to the fallopian tube to fertilize the female egg.

On Reproductive Organs

Prostate

The prostate is at the lower part of the bladder surrounding the urethra and produces a large portion of the fluid and chemicals that make up the semen. Also, the prostate can constrict to prevent urine and semen from flowing at the wrong time.

Membranous urethra

The membranous urethra or intermediate part of the male urethra is the shortest, least dilatable, and narrower than other parts of the urethra. It lies within the urogenital diaphragm. This membrane acts as a sensory valve that allows urine and semen to flow to the urethra during ejaculation and urination. It is surrounded by the sphincter fibers and terminates at the Cowper's glands.

Cowper's Glands

A pair of Cowper's glands reside beneath the prostate and in front of the anus. The Cowper's glands produce a thin alkaline fluid that lubricates the urethra and neutralizes the acid left in the urethra after urination. The slimy fluid enters the urethra during sexual arousal before ejaculation to prepare the urethra for semen flow.

Semen

Semen is the fluid produced by males during sexual intercourse. It contains sperm and chemicals that make it thick, sticky, and slimy. These chemicals allow it to remain within the vagina after sex and neutralize the vagina's acidic environment.

Naked Compassion

In healthy adult males, semen contains millions of sperms.

Urethra

The urethra is a long muscular tube that runs from the bladder to the orifice of the penis. It also runs through the prostate. Semen from the ejaculatory tube and urine from the bladder also pass through the urethra.

Corpora Cavernosa

The corpora cavernosa is a pair of sponge-like tissue that lie along the penis shaft and fill with blood during an erection.

Corpus Spongiosa

The corpus Spongiosa are the soft tissue that runs under the corpus cavernosa. It extends from the bulb of the penis to the far end. And continuous with the crown of the penis through the center of which runs the urethra. When the corpus cavernosa becomes hard to support the penis, they remains relatively soft to hold the urethra open to allow the semen to pass quickly.

Penis

The penis is a male organ that hangs on the upper part of the scrotum and underneath the umbilicus. The penis is roughly cylindrical and contains the urethra and the orifice of the penis. Massive tissue around the penis allows blood to fill it and get it erect. When the penis gets erect, it increases in size and becomes turgid. The penis delivers semen to the vagina during sexual intercourse. Besides, the penis also allows urine to flow through the urethra to the outside of the body.

On Reproductive Organs

Female Reproductive Organs

*I hear men talk about it and ask why the fascination. It's
frustrating, a little voice tells me; they crave the home they once
lived in and want to go back for a visit. It all makes sense now*

✳✳✳

Although this book is about preventing sperm from getting
into a woman's vagina, learning a few things about a woman's
reproductive system is essential to understanding how sperm
moves inside a woman's vagina. You will learn how the female
reproductive system makes a woman's egg and transports it to
the fallopian tube, where conception occurs. So here's the
layman's description of the essential structure of the organs that
make up the female reproductive system:

Ovaries

Two small glands, the ovaries, reside in the pelvic body
cavity along the uterus's upper left and right sides. Ovaries
produce female sex hormones such as estrogen and
progesterone. Ovaries also produce ova, the female gametes
commonly known as the egg. The oocyte cells that slowly
develop throughout a woman's early life and reach maturity after
puberty contain the ova. Each month during ovulation, the ovary
releases a mature egg into the fallopian tube, where the sperm
may fertilize it before reaching the uterus.

Naked Compassion

Fallopian Tubes

Fallopian tubes are a pair of muscular tubes covered in cilia. It extends from left to right on the upper corners of the uterus to the ovaries' edge. The fallopian tubes end in a funnel-like structure called the infundibulum, covered by small finger-like fimbriae. The Fimbriae hang over the ovaries to pick up released ova and carry them into the infundibulum for transport to the uterus.

Uterus

The uterus is a hollow muscular pear-like organ on the urinary bladder's upper backside. It also connects to the two fallopian tubes on the top end and the vagina through the cervix. The uterus is supportive and surrounds the developing fetus; hence, it is the womb.

Vagina

The vagina lies between the vulva and the uterus. It connects the two through the cervix, serving as a receptacle for sperm during sexual intercourse and a passageway for childbirth.

Vulva

The entire exterior of the female genitalia is called the vulva. It includes the vestibule, labia majora, labia minora, the urethra orifice, and the clitoris.

PART 8

NAKED
COMPASSION

On Smart Pullout Guide

*I've learned that people will forget what you said and what you did,
but people will never forget how you made them feel.*

~ Maya Angelou

On Smart Pullout Guide

Behind the Feeling

✳✳✳

In this part, you will learn how the organs that make up the reproductive system work together to produce sperm, transport it and store it for ejaculation. You will know how the male reproductive system converts sperm to semen. And what makes the semen capable of swimming upstream to the female fallopian tubes. Besides, you will learn how your nervous system's sensitivities and sexual pleasure change along the way until ejaculation occurs—internally before semen gets out of the body through the penis. At this point, I have to say:

The "Smart Pullout" is a standard of living. To make it a way of life, you must practice it persistently, diligently, and with compassion. If not to prevent unwanted pregnancy, then do it for respect, appreciation, and a sense of caring for the woman you love.

Keep the Carnal Senses Active

Talk sense to a fool, and he calls you foolish.

~ Euripides, The Bacchae

A successful pullout depends on various factors such as

Naked Compassion

age, health, biology, and how the following carnal senses affect sexual pleasure:

Touch and Feel

The sense of touch and feel emanates from playful, gentle, caressing wonderingly, exploring with fingertips, and coming into contact with the face and other body parts. It creates sexual excitement that usually leads to a sweet surrender, which signals the desire for sperm ejaculation.

Smell

The smell comes from the pleasant odor or scent that creates sexual desire and often stimulates the reproductive system's nerve endings. Naturally, women grasp the spirit of smell far more than men; hence, it is common to find sensuous perfume in a woman's home by the nightstand or bathroom cabinet. In short, a sweet aroma elevates sexual desires.

Taste

This is the act of becoming acquainted with by experience and ascertaining its flavor by taking a small quantity into the mouth, which often leads to kissing. Sometimes it comes from a curious imagination that what looks or smells must also taste good, so it gets the blood flowing to the desired areas.

Voice

The sound a mate makes during sexual activities, which, if suggestive and interactive, can enhance sexual pleasure. Verbal interaction is a powerful fuel for sexual energy. Understanding each other's tone helps the female know when to move her

On Smart Pullout Guide

vagina away and out of her mate's penis' reach. And in so doing, it contributes to the success of the pullout. This point is worth emphasizing. Believe it or not, vocal interaction is the most overlooked part of the sexual exercise that often causes mates to screw up the pullout.

Imagery

Imagery is the ornate or heightened mental appearance of a mate's beauty, look, and figure, which often produces a particular effect (such as a distinctive emotional appeal or loving euphoria) during the peak of sexual intercourse shortly before ejaculation. As I've experienced most of the time, when the sperm inside the ejaculatory duct becomes semen, the female looks the most beautiful she can look—a prelude to climax. "IT HELPS TO KEEP YOUR EYES OPEN."

Presence

Presence is the silent mental and physical state of being in the same place as someone precious—not separated by an inch, barrier, or time. It leads to a disarming sense of gratitude and satisfaction before ejaculation. For a moment, we become aware of how close we are to our mates and feel grateful. In essence, the absence of presence signifies an unsatisfactory sexual session. Delightful foreplay is a part of the game. Indeed, foreplay warms up the entire reproductive nervous system and gets the blood and sperm moving.

Keep Your Eyes Open

Having sex under the light of pleasing softness, color, and brightness allows mates to see each other's faces and is as vital

Naked Compassion

as audible signaling of the orgasm or imminent cum 's arrival. In most cases, during sexual intercourse, when a man or woman is about to cum, there is a profound change in their facial expression. So the ability to observe this change, which often takes the form of looking as handsome or beautiful as they could to looking like somebody in pain or merely making a funny face, helps mates discern the point of ejaculation and exercise the pullout successfully.

With all the information and knowledge you gained from the preceding passages, it is time to shed your doubts about the "smart pullout" pregnancy prevention technique and get to work. You can follow the guide, put that knowledge into use, relieve your mate of that nagging stress and agony from unwanted pregnancy fears, and experience sex like you never imagined.

Arousal to Ejaculation

*It is not the brains that matter most but that which guides them —
the character, the heart, generous qualities, and progressive ideas.*

~ Fyodor Dostoevsky

This passage is the Smart pullout users' guide. It describes how sperm moves from its production to ejaculation, why the level of your sexual pleasure changes when sperm reaches vital sex organs, and most importantly, the right time to pull the penis out of the vagina.

1. As you foreplay, blood rush to the erectile spongy

On Smart Pullout Guide

corpora cavernosa. Now the penis gets hard and erect, and the man feels the desire for sex and urges for immediate intromission into the vagina.

2. The brain signals the epididymis to start sperm migration through the vas deferens. Then sperm migrating into vas deferens displaces those already stored in it.

3. The vas deferens begin to transport sperm stored in it towards the ampulla. Sperm passing through the vas deferens is not yet motile—able to swim, so smooth muscle tissue in the walls of the vas deferens contract in waves and slowly move sperm towards the ampulla.

This process is known as peristalsis, which causes sex to feel good.

4. After sperm enters the ampulla, the fresh sperm pushes the sperm previously stored in it into the ejaculatory duct.

5. The ejaculatory duct signals the prostate and the seminal vesicle to secrete fluids to convert the sperm to semen.

Sex begins to feel so good the man scurries and with thrust.

6. Next, the fluid from the seminal vesicles and the prostate combine at the ejaculatory duct and transforms the sperm into semen—**thicker slimier juice.**

7. The mixing of sperm and chemicals is a crucial point. The thick semen causes downward pressure on the urogenital diaphragm.

Naked Compassion

This process forces the penis and the corona to become very sensitive.

8. If the mates have engaged in good foreplay or the sexual intercourse has been well done and lasted long enough to arouse the female, the vagina gets wet.

The vagina and penis become extremely sensitive, and the vestibule becomes tender. And now, the sexual pleasure becomes overwhelming.

9. Those who practice the "smart pullout" persistently often discover their avid fondness for sexual delight comes from this immersed flesh-to-flesh state where the penis moves viscously in and out of the wet vagina as the vestibule hugs the corona.

It is a feeling that fosters an appreciation of that particular person from whom you derive your sexual pleasure—that you will never experience with a condom.

At this point, the membranous urethra senses sperm entering the urogenital diaphragm and producing overwhelming sexual pleasure.

10. By definition, orgasm is the sexual climax, where you nut or ejaculate. Stated differently, it is the point at

On Smart Pullout Guide

which sexual pleasure is optimal and overwhelming to the senses.

Caution, you have less than one second before losing control. For the most part, this is the point and time when most people screw up, thinking there's more fun left. No! This is it! The ejaculation has occurred, and the reproductive system has already donated to the various hormone-producing organs. So here is what you must do:

Scream, cry, yell, or shout, "I'm Cumming" and immediately pull your penis out of the vagina. All that is left is the transportation of the semen to its final destination.

Why Audible?

Here are two answers to this question:

1. Yelling or crying slows the forward momentum and creates a counterforce that moves you backward, away from your mate. So, it would help if you were vocal.

2. Screaming lets the female know when ejaculation is imminent, allowing her to push the male away from her.

Naked Compassion

Summary

The following is the summary of the Smart pullout users' guide that emphasizes the concept of sperm flow and position awareness, which is worth remembering during sexual intercourse to make the "smart pullout" successful. These facts manifest in the form of sexual pleasure, heartbeat, and sensitivity of the body parts:

- As you foreplay, blood rush to the erectile spongy corpora cavernosa. Now the penis gets hard and erect, and the man feels the desire for sex and urges for immediate intromission into the vagina.

- The brain signals the epididymis to start sperm migration through the vas deferens. Then sperm migrating into vas deferens displaces those already stored in it.

- The vas deferens begin to transport sperm stored in it towards the ampulla. Sperm passing through the vas deferens is not yet motile—able to swim, so smooth muscle tissue in the walls of the vas deferens contract in waves and slowly move sperm towards the ampulla.

- The Cowper's gland produces wetness to neutralize urine left in the urethra after urination and prepare it for sperm flow.

- The sperm arriving at the ampulla displace those already stored in it, causing them to move into the ejaculatory duct.

On Smart Pullout Guide

- The fluid from the seminal vesicles and the prostate combine at the ejaculatory duct and transforms the sperm into semen.

- The mixing of sperm and chemicals is a crucial point. The thick semen causes downward pressure on the urogenital diaphragm.

- If the mates have engaged in good foreplay or the sexual intercourse has been well done and lasted long enough to arouse the female, the vagina gets wet.

- At this point, the sexual pleasure comes from this immersed flesh-to-flesh state, where the penis moves viscously in and out of the wet vagina as the vestibule hugs the corona.

- The membranous urethra senses semen entering the urogenital diaphragm, producing overwhelming sexual pleasure.

- At this moment, sexual pleasure overwhelms the senses. Realistically, the male has less than one second to pull the penis from the vagina.

- Ejaculation has already occurred internally, and the mates have reaped the full benefits of sex.

- Your pullout is successful if you move your penis away from the vagina and the vulva and watch the sperm arrive.

It may seem easy in words or on paper; however, it is a different story in practice, so you need training and help from an expert. For further help and guidance, refer to the section titled Resources.

Naked Compassion

Male Pre-cum Wetness

Most people confuse semen and pre-cum wetness during sexual intercourse. When you arouse the male reproductive system sexually, the Cowper's glands secrete a thin alkaline fluid into the urethra to lubricate the urethra. The juice also neutralizes the acid from urine remaining in the urethra after urination. This fluid enters the urethra during sexual intercourse before ejaculation to prepare the urethra for semen flow. According to research, pre-cum does not have the essential markers that give sperm the capability of swimming upstream to hunt for the female egg along the fallopian tube.

Female Pre-Cum Wetness

It is natural for a woman to have vaginal discharge, and it's normal for a woman's vagina to become "wet." This wetness lubricates her vagina when sexually aroused.

I came across the above quote when I was researching this book. Why should you know? The female cervix produces mucus, which lines the vagina and expels it as discharge. During sexual foreplay, veins in a woman's vaginal tissues dilate and fill with blood, gradually making the whole area feel full. In the vagina, this swelling creates a "sweating reaction," producing a fluid that causes the vaginal lips to get wet—often an early sign that a woman is sexually aroused. This fluid wets the entrance to the vagina, making penetration easier and pleasurable.

On Smart Pullout Guide

Worksheets

✳✳✳

This section contains the essential materials from the preceding parts. Below is a worksheet for you to practice with and test your knowledge of the Smart pullout until you can name every vital sex organ and aspect of the reproductive system accurately and the sperm flow pathways from the epididymis to the penis:

Practice Quiz 1

Assign numbers to the following regarding the order of sperm production, flow, position, and release from the body. Assign the letter "D" to glands that perform contributory functions such as donating chemicals that transform sperm into semen or neutralizing acid left in the urethra after urination.

__) Prostate
__) Ampulla
__) Epididymis
__) Testes
__) Vas or ductus Deferens
__) Seminal vesicles
__) Ejaculatory Duct
__) Penis
__) Cowper's Glands
__) Membranous Urethra

Naked Compassion

Practice Quiz 2

For the following organs, enter "F" for female, "M" for male and "B" for both:

_) Prostate
_) Ovaries
_) Ampulla
_) Epididymis
_) Clitoris
_) Testes
_) Vas Deferens
_) Vulva
_) Seminal vesicles
_) Fallopian Tubes
_) Ejaculatory Duct
_) Uterus
_) Penis
_) Cowper's Glands
_) Vagina
_) Membranous Urethra
_) Cervix
_) Urethra orifice

Practice Quiz 3

It is essential to be aware of the changes in your sexual pleasure and why during intercourse. The following questions will help you master and Identify the sperm position during sexual intercourse. You can improve your mastery of the sperm flow and position awareness by answering the following

On Smart Pullout Guide

questions:

1. What is the first thing that happens when a man is sexually excited?

   _____

2. Name the organ responsible for male erection

   _____

3. What is the function of Epididymis?

   _____

4. What is peristalsis?

   _____

5. Identify the position of sperm at the onset of sexual pleasure.

   _____

6. What is the function of vas deferens?

   _____

7. Name the enlarged portion of the vas deferens.

   _____

8. At what point does vas deferens end?

   _____

9. What is the difference between sperm and semen?

   _____

10. Name the two organs that produce the fluid that

Naked Compassion

converts sperm to semen.

_____

11. At what point during sexual intercourse does sex start to feel good?

_____

12. Inside which duct is sperm converted to semen.

_____

13. At what point during sexual intercourse does sexual pleasure overwhelm the senses?

_____

14. Which organ produces the fluid that neutralizes acid left in the urethra after urination?

_____

15. What is pre-cum?

_____

16. When semen reaches this membrane, you have less than one second to pull your penis from the vagina. Name the membrane.

_____

17. What is the function of the Cowper's glands?

_____

18. How can you tell you've had worry-free sex?

_____

On Smart Pullout Guide

19. This duct stores sperm before sexual activities.
Name the duct.

_____

20. Sperm travels a long distance from its production to ejaculation. What is the name of this tube through which it travels?

Practice Quiz 4

What is the best way to guard against sexually transmitted infections?

Answer for Quiz 1

D) Prostate
4) Ampulla
2) Epididymis
1) Testes
3) vas or ductus Deferens
D) Seminal vesicles
5) Ejaculatory Duct
7) Penis
D) Cowper's Glands
6) Membranous Urethra

Answer for Quiz 2

M) Prostate
F) Ovaries

Naked Compassion

M) Ductus Ampulla

M) Epididymis

F) Clitoris

M) Testes

M) vas Deferens

F) Vulva

M) Seminal vesicles

F) Fallopian Tubes

M) Ejaculatory Duct

F) Uterus

M) Penis

M) Cowper's or Bulbourethral Glands

F) Vagina

M) Membranous Urethra

F) Cervix

B) Urethra orifice

Answer for Quiz 3

1.
_____ Corpora cavernosa fills with blood__

2.
_____ Corpora cavernosa _____

3.
___It stores fresh sperm until it matures___

4.
__Natural movement by successive waves of
Involuntary contraction within the hollow muscular
Structure of vas deferens___

5.
_____Ampulla_____

On Smart Pullout Guide

6.
__It carries sperm from the epididymis to the ampulla __

7.
_____Ampulla____

8.
___Ampulla __

9.
___Semen contains proteins, mucus, fructose, and Alkaline ph. Sperm does not___

10.
___Prostate and seminal vesicle ___

11.
___When the sperm enters the ejaculatory duct __

12.
___In the ejaculatory duct __

13.
__When semen presses on the membranous urethra_

14.
___ Cowper's gland ___

15.
__Fluid is added to the urethra to neutralize the acid left inside the track after urination ___

16.
_____Membranous urethra____

17.
__To add fluid to the urethra to neutralize acid left Inside the track and prepare it for semen flow __

18.
___When the penis is entirely outside the vagina and away from the vulva before cum rushes out ___

19.

Naked Compassion

20.

_____Ampulla_____

_____Vas Deferens _____

Answer for Quiz 4

You and your mate should undergo a blood test at the beginning of your relationship and periodically ensure both are STI-free and have sex only with each other.

If you answered all the questions correctly, Congratulations! You are now on your way to becoming adept in the act of the Smart pull unwanted pregnancy prevention technique

If you did not, don't worry; keep reading and practicing or, if necessary, refer to the passage captioned "Resources" for further help.

Resources

We have designed an online training program to assist NAKED COMPASSION readers and everybody interested in the STI and Smart Pullout pregnancy prevention techniques. For further information regarding this training program, please visit https://www.smartpullout.com/

Other Books By Chuks I. Ndukwe

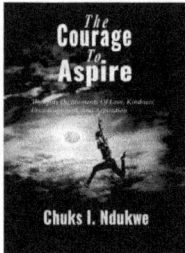

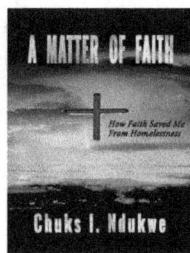

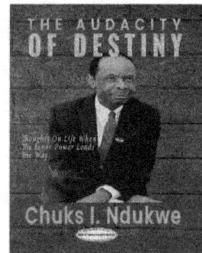

www.ingramcontent.com/pod-product-compliance
Lightning Source LLC
Chambersburg PA
CBHW030250030426
42336CB00009B/322